HOMO
SAPIENS

Imperfectus

HOMO
HEIDELBERGENESIS

HOMO
NEANDERTHALENSIS

HOMO
FLORIENSIS

HOMO
~~SAPIENS~~

Imperfectus

A Reconstruction of Behavioural Science and Psychiatry

ROBERT BUGLER
F.R.C.PSYCH., M.R.C.G.P.

This concept is theoretical; it should not be used to advance any new therapeutic approach in the absence of properly supervised research.

First published in Great Britain in 2023 by
Robert Bugler, in partnership with whitefox publishing

www.wearewhitefox.com

ISBN 978-1-915635-00-6
Also available as an eBook
ISBN 978-1-915635-33-4

Cover design by Simon Levy
Typeset by Jill Sawyer
Project management by whitefox

CONTENTS

PREAMBLE

I have hoped for many years that someone more talented than I would reach similar conclusions and set out the following concept more capably.

The concept is an evolution of behaviour, of response to change from elemental phenomena to human disorders, to our mental illnesses.

I have no talent for writing, and even less for communicating, but I am driven to publish the work by a conviction that it contributes to our knowledge of human behaviour and the psychological disorders that burden many of us.

INTRODUCTION

This work arose from frustration that my field, psychiatry, has not made the same dramatic advances that medicine and surgery have achieved in the past half-century. In addition, as a child psychiatrist I have been dismayed that the profession has been unable to account for the peculiar vulnerability of children and the persistence of damage into adulthood, of 'Adverse Childhood Events', particularly sexual abuse.

There is no scientific framework for childhood fragilities and consequences. Without a scientific foundation new theories and different forms of management are taken up, pursued, and dropped and quickly replaced. It confuses parents and teachers and can affect children's lives.

A defining feature of psychiatry and of my own sub-specialty, child psychiatry, has been one of continuous fluctuation through changing philosophical interpretations of mental disorder and its management. The transience is demonstrated by the eleven revisions of The International Classification of Mental Disorders[1] that have taken place since formal classification was first introduced in the early 1960s.

A logical evidence-based system remains elusive.

Before retiring I endeavoured to interest colleagues in what I believed to be a stasis of the field and was treated as an oddball, to be a little indulged or avoided. I learnt to keep my convictions

---

[1]   https://www.ncbi.nlm.nih.gov/pmc/articles/PMC6313247/

to myself, but in moving out of active involvement and happening upon Thomas Kuhn's *The Structure of Scientific Revolutions*, my conviction that the specialty needed reconstruction was renewed.

In seeking a new approach, I reached a conclusion that the relative failure of psychiatry to progress had occurred through the absence of an evolution and system of behaviour, of organic **response to change**. In short, psychiatry's relative stasis is a failure of behavioural science, not that of psychiatrists.

It also appeared to be obvious to me that human susceptibility to psychiatric disorder coincided with our evolution from earlier primates and our dramatic increase in intelligence. An increase that showed no evidence of being accompanied by an advanced decision-making facility.

The effect can be compared to a canteen chef being asked to provide a Michelin service with inevitable breakdown.

FUNDAMENTAL
RESPONSE TO CHANGE

Responding to change is as fundamental an organic need as metabolizing food and offloading unwanted by-products. Metabolism has a series of organs to carry out the necessary processes, these organs contributing to a system that we label the metabolic or digestive system. We have other systems, including the muscular-skeletal system, which should be labelled the mobility system, and the cardio-vascular or logistics system.

Our brain and nerves are organs of the response to change system and like our other systems, the form in which the system functions can only be elucidated by identifying the elemental phenomena and their evolution from that point. This work offers a rational evolution from simple responses, through to human behaviour and susceptibility to psychological disorders when their characteristics become rational.

These days it is usual to give a warning that material may offend. Through one aspect or another, the subversive concept takes every reader out of their comfort zone. It discomforts me, but if it leads to a rethinking that eases the misery of psychiatric illness and children's vulnerability, it will have been worthwhile.

* * *

It is difficult to communicate the reconfiguration of any field. The task is aggravated in this work as the accepted labels for emotions and motivations do not coincide with the reconfiguration. In endeavouring to keep replacement neologisms to an absolute minimum, simplistic terms and analogies have frequently been employed.

RESPONSE TO CHANGE – BEHAVIOUR

In fundamental character, external change is either benign or adverse. When it is benign, organic life is open to the environment, exchanging material with it. When it is adverse, organic life withdraws from the environment and inhibits exchange.

In this work, responding to a benign condition is referred to as '**apertic**' after the Latin 'open door'; withdrawing from the environment is '**recedic**'.

Behaviour 'response to change' has steadily evolved from that point, primarily through the gradual modification of the initially polarized perceptions and responses.

* * *

The elemental responses are evident in our own behaviour. When others around us are hospitable to us, friendly, we are outgoing and can with incontinently loud voice and physical gestures become intrusive upon bystanders, upon any who are not part of the group. We are intrusive upon the immediate environment. We enjoy the emotion that we have at those times.

When we are in company and those around us are unwilling to relate to us, who are in effect rejecting us, it is inhospitable and we self-contain, we restrict our presence. We are uncomfortable.

Our variable levels of emotions have many adjectives to describe them. Adolescents have acute emotions and find the available terms inadequate to describe the intensity that they experience. Consequently, every generation coins a new vocabulary to convey the near overwhelming adolescent emotions. Recently, in 2022, 'banging', 'sick' and others.

In that context, interviewers constantly press interviewees to say how they are feeling after a significant event, seemingly in the hope of an extraordinary new revelation. The reality is that we have two emotions, we are **ill at ease** when we are compelled by the environment to be **recedic** and we are **at greater ease** when the environment allows us to be **apertic**, both only altering in intensity.

It is not only the company we keep that makes the environment benign for us. We are also influenced by the climate and the many different sensory experiences that we enjoy: food, music, the state of our homes, can all affect our mood. It is possible that there are other qualities of the environment such as atmospheric pressure, that unconsciously influence us too.

We are for much of the day, mildly apertic or mildly recedic.

BIOLOGICAL LAWS

For the past century, and following the work of Charles Darwin and Gregor Mendel, the almost universal presumption has been that species have evolved through genetic change filtered by Darwinian 'selection of the fittest' – in short, that every physical and behavioural characteristic is in place because it contributes to survival of the individual or of the species.

In this concept, the evolution and nature of behaviour, of organic 'response to change', are modified by biological laws as well as the Darwinian formula. One consequence is that behaviour can be interpreted in other contexts than that of being directed towards personal or species survival.

The protocols that are allocated law-like status are not personal inventions but well-recognized and accepted phenomena. They are almost as inescapable as the laws of physics.

THE FIRST BIOLOGICAL 'LAW': THE NEED TO EXPERIENCE A CHANGING ENVIRONMENT

Every tissue or organ and every organism needs to function, to be exercised from time to time, to maintain its viability. The phenomenon is evident when the blood or nerve supply to a muscle is cut and not restored. In that circumstance the muscle ceases to function and it is gradually replaced by collagen, a scar-like fibrous tissue.

The 'law' also applies to recedism and apertism – environmental changes can ensure that both are exercised. But many environments are relatively stable, so consequently unicellular life evolved flagella and cilia that facilitate movement and provide the necessary changing experience. Halophilic bacteria in the Dead Sea, for example, achieve change with gas vacuoles that float them to the surface. The purpose is debated because the need to experience change is not recognized as a vital exercise or behaviour by the academic community.[2]

Both activities are satisfied in most animals and in our own lives by the diurnal rotation of night and day, between being generally active, apertic, during the day, and self-contained, recedic, during the night. Some species reverse the alternation and are most active during the night.

SECOND BIOLOGICAL 'LAW': CELLULAR OSCILLATION

All cells oscillate.

Oscillation is little considered in biological research and has not been integrated into behavioural science, but it influences our behaviour.

Its inclusion in this work fulfils Thomas Kuhn's observation that every successful scientific reorientation integrates material from another science.

The presence and characteristics of oscillation as an essential component of cellular physiology were established by Brian Goodwin (1931–2009) whilst working at MIT in 1965. His paper 'A Statistical Mechanics of Temporal Organization in Cells' was

---

[2] Department of Plant and Environmental Sciences, The Alexander Silberman Institute of Life Sciences, The Hebrew University of Jerusalem, 91904, Jerusalem, *Israel Life* 2013, 3(1), 1-20.
A few extremely halophilic Archaea [...] possess gas vesicles that bestow buoyancy on the cells [...] existing studies failed to provide clear evidence for their possible function. This paper summarizes the current status of the different theories why gas vesicles may provide a selective advantage to some halophilic micro-organisms.

submitted at a symposium of the Society for Experimental Biology and published in its journal, No 18, 1965, pp 301–326.

In his paper, Professor Goodwin demonstrated that:

i)   all cells oscillate,
ii) the activity facilitated homeostasis,
iii) when oscillation is interrupted cells do not survive,
iv) cellular oscillation adjusts to stimuli: in an equable environment, it is a fine vibration.

When the environment alters, both the rhythm of oscillation and biochemical balance are amplified, inducted more powerfully to prevent internal function from being disorganized.[3]

Whatever process initiated cellular oscillation, once it developed, it had a vital role. Oscillation, however, has the equivalent of a life of its own. It is difficult to modify, and just as any cacophonous noise affects us, it intrudes upon everything in its vicinity.

The influence of oscillation on behaviour is set out later in this work.

THIRD BIOLOGICAL 'LAW': ECONOMY OR EFFICIENT USE OF RESOURCES

Organic life is economic in use of material and energy resources; any species that fails to use resources efficiently is replaced by another that does.

---

[3]   The presence of oscillation in bacteria and the cells of living tissues is established, but the following may more clearly reveal the close association between oscillation and physiological processes. From *Scientific American* 'Ask the Experts', 3 April 2006: 'Why do cats purr?' Cats purr during both inhalation and exhalation with a consistent pattern and frequency between 25 and 150 Hertz. Various investigators have shown that the sound frequencies in this range improve bone density and promote healing.
ALSO High frequency oscillation in patients with acute lung injury (ARDS) reduces hospital or 30-day mortality and improves oxygenation. *BMJ*, 2010; 340: c2327 doi: 10.1136/bmj.c2327

As five to ten per cent of the calories we ingest is spent on maintaining our vital body temperature (around 37°C), we try to be economic in expending our own energy; we insulate ourselves with clothes and heat our houses.

FOURTH BIOLOGICAL 'LAW': HOMEOSTASIS

Cellular homeostasis was established as a vital physiological attribute by Claude Bernard (1813–1878), sometimes referred to as the 'father' of physiology. His axiom, translated from French, was: 'all vital mechanisms, varied as they are, have only one object: that of preserving constant the conditions of life.' The American physiologist Walter Bradford Cannon (1871–1945) introduced the term homeostasis to describe this innate constancy. (*Encyclopaedia Britannica*)

To maintain homeostasis as economically as possible, we seek and enjoy a comfortable homeostatic external environment. It is at odds with the need to experience change.

COMPETITION

Competition is an extension of the need to experience change. When change is neutralized by achieving a benign stable condition, game playing, winning and losing, provide a stimulating variation. Winning terminates a challenge as effectively as losing, the successful 'game' is indefinitely preserving a dynamic balance.

It is reflected in the difference between playing noughts and crosses (tic-tac-toe) and playing chess. Whilst the former very rapidly ceases to retain interest, playing chess can be addictive.

THE THREE ERAS IN
THE EVOLUTION OF
BEHAVIOUR

First era. Unicellular: maintaining an intact physiology through violent climatic and geological change of the physical environment.
Second era. Multicellular: survival response to the presence of prey and predators, to other species.
Third era. Human: establishing personal self-respect in exchange with and in response to our own species.

UNICELLULAR ERA

When the first cells arose from congregations of organic molecules approximately 3,500 million years ago, the environment was subject to violent geological and climatic changes. Bacterial physiology was fragile and constantly threatened by disruption, even complete dissolution by extreme change. Bacteria developed the ability to virtually separate from the environment to secure their physiology and ensure self-preservation by becoming spores. The spore's thick coat insulates the inner cytoplasm from extreme temperatures, acids and alkalis.

Cultivation of unicellular life in the laboratory demonstrates that primitive cells separate from both potentially lethal and excessively benign circumstances in physically different actions but with similar results:

1. In extremely adverse circumstances the cell becomes an impervious spore and divides into multiple particles inside a thickened external coat.
2. In consistently benign environments, primitive cells grow and split into two: 'parthenogenesis'. The process continues through multiple generations, but, ultimately, and in this concept
    i)   through the biological need to periodically exercise every function,
    ii)   including that of ability to separate from the environment,
    iii) continuous generation ends in sporulation.

Human reactions follow a similar pattern. When an extreme event (fire, explosion) has arisen, we separate from it before compulsively reporting the experience to many others, sharing it with as many as possible, and as soon as possible.

In the most extreme benign circumstances, the very rich separate, retreat from the community and subsequently (like bacteria, much later) 'spreading the excess benign' by becoming philanthropic.

Lethal Events

Potentially lethal events provoke an involuntary, reflex-like separation in human lives. The separation is achieved either by: (i) withdrawing, absenting oneself from the situation, accompanied by fear – or (ii) aggressive destruction, removal, 'taking out', of whatever has been experienced as the significant threat, accompanied by anger.

Some separation responses are inherent. We react in knee-jerk, reflex response when we are exposed to devastating explosion or fire. In those events, parents will separate, rush from the scene, involuntarily deserting their children. Birds flee from hawk-like shapes in the sky without ever having been attacked by one. Many species avoid snakes, and many humans separate from animals that have unusual movement such as spiders and crabs.

In the most extreme, sudden, adverse events, we separate as totally as possible from the external environment. Our intestinal and urinary tracts evacuate any unincorporated material: we vomit, become incontinent, or both.

Every road accident can have lethal consequences, a separation response may be provoked, either a powerful impulse to remove oneself, to fly from the event, or to remove the cause – the other driver – and road rage (aggressive destruction) results.

* * *

It is logical that severe PTSD (post-traumatic stress disorder) occurs when a life-threatening experience cannot be responded to, either by acting in separation from a lethal threat or by taking steps to remove it, especially in isolated circumstances.

Soldiers in the First World War were executed when a PTSD-like condition provoked their refusal to return to the front line, to fight. In some cases, those affected had shown bravery more than once, in retrieving fallen comrades whilst under fire for example, but after being buried by shell fire on further occasion, they refused to advance, to re-enter the battlefield. Rather than risk returning to the intolerable paralysed experience, where neither form of separation can be attempted, they chose to be executed, to commit suicide.

In all cases of PTSD, subsequent random experiences, such as conversations, pictures or events, that recall the episode must stimulate 'don't go near again', an acute emotion we label 'anxiety'. The phenomenon suggests that our decision-making facility dictates: 'do not enter into the impossible, the unresolvable, again'. In that context, and technically, the hippocampus, part of the decision-making hind brain, forms and reconstructs relational memory necessary for remembering arbitrary associations between objects or events.

In suicide we remove ourselves or separate from the intolerable, in murder we remove the unacceptable.

Tears
Both extremely happy and extremely sad events can provoke one universal 'reflex separation' response. Our eyes 'water' to physically

separate from invading grit, but they can also water – cry – when we are reunited with close relatives we have been parted from for a long time – and when we lose them in death.

Extreme Events

Extreme events provoke separation, or a gesture of separation, from the material or social environment. We experience emotional arousal when we must make decisions about the best action to take. The emotional arousal is alleviated when a decision is made, whether it is to act apertically or recedically. It is essential for the anxiety/arousal to be dissipated by one path or another for arousal to return to emotional equanimity and physiological homeostasis. If arousal persists, we are unable to judge, to make accurate decisions about new events, in any persistent emotional state, be it anxiety, misery or fury.

We are fortunate when a night's sleep with REM (dreaming) mitigates the emotional arousal of extreme adverse or benign events. There is an extensive list of adjectives attached to our emotions, to the arousal that we experience when there has been a significant event. The reality is that differentiating emotional descriptions – terror, triumph and the whole lexicon of those adjectives – are artificial fallacies. The arousal of terror and triumph are similar, they can differ in intensity, but it is the event that we are passing through that gives us a label for the emotion.

A FURTHER STAGE OF UNICELLULAR LIFE

In the preliminary stages of organic life, simple cells functioned by elemental responses to change. They evolved to more complex entities with multiple and contradictory attributes, including apertism, recedism, maintenance of homeostasis, oscillation, a need to experience change in the environment, and the efficient use of resources.

The attributes can be compared to musicians each striving to bring the sound of their own instrument to the fore, to voice their contributions and their needs.

Then there was a vacancy for a director to rotate activity, according to functional necessity and in relation to fluctuation of the external environment. The role was filled by a third parasite-like molecule that invaded the cell to become the nucleus. In being parasitic it created a hospitable environment for itself, it 'managed' the internal environment of the cell by having an 'awareness' of internal and external conditions and in reinforcing the stable internal state, the cellular 'homeostasis'. It was advantageous through the efficiency that it introduced for the host cell, and the relationship between the three tissues, the cytoplasm, the cell wall and the nucleus, became mutually dependent.

In making decisions, the nucleus – and eventually our hind brains – need to combine:

i)   Weighing different degrees of adverse and benign qualities of the environment – like the fulcrum of simple weighing scales.
ii) Organizing the response at several layers like an orchestral conductor.
iii) Managing physiology like a laboratory chemist.

OSCILLATION – AND ITS EFFECT UPON BEHAVIOUR

The properties of oscillating bodies are so precise that they are only defined as mathematical formulae. Without 'written' laws, it is difficult for the lay person, including myself, to understand and apply the effects of oscillation. The following is a personal attempt to represent some of the mathematical formulae of oscillation as working models.

There are three common examples of oscillating bodies: the pendulums of 19th-century clocks, the desk toys – or Newton pendulums – with multiple bobs or weights, and that of children oscillating backwards and forwards on a swing.

All three are useful models in identifying the integration of oscillation with behaviour.

Oscillation is not only vital to cellular life, it influences our behaviour,

i)   as the foundation of biological rhythms,
ii) it modifies the speed and momentum with which we respond to an event and
iii) dramatically influences our relationships.

The relevant properties integrated into behaviour are:

CHRONOMETER. Precise timing, a regular pulse that can be compared to a metronome that assists musicians in maintaining the correct rhythm.

ENERGY. Potential and kinetic energy which influence both perception of and response to change in the environment.

SYNCHRONY. Synchrony between oscillating bodies which influences relationships.

CHRONOMETER-LIKE REGULAR PULSATION

Our complex physiology is dependent upon biological rhythms that could not exist without the underlying clock-like resource of cellular oscillation:

Biological Rhythms

Many physiological processes can be compared to machines in a factory. Efficient machines undertake more than one task and they manage it by fulfilling one 'responsibility' before rotating to another.

We have at least 241 biological rhythms operating within us; we are usually only aware of menstruation, cardiac, respiratory and sleep rhythms.

'Humans and other animals have genetically based biological clocks that are present in individual cells resulting in semi-autonomous oscillators in many peripheral tissues that can be coordinated by the suprachiasmic nucleus in the anterior hypothalamus[4].'[5]

Possibly because it is the most physiologically integrated, the menstrual cycle may affect emotions more than any other rhythm.[6]

In everyone's life, a common change of mood is caused by

---

[4]   The hypothalamus is part of the hind brain.
[5]   Koukkari and Sothern, *Introducing Biological Rhythms* (Springer Science, 2006) p 433.
[6]   Louann Brizendine was struck by the extent to which the female brain is shaped by dramatic changes in hormonal chemistry, driving a woman's behaviour and creating her reality. Butler-Bowden, Tim, ed., *50 Psychology Classics* (Nicholas Brealey Publishing, 2012) p 53.

high insulin secretion in the afternoon. It reduces blood glycogen, making us less alert and less amenable to others. We may not recognize that we are being ill-natured, but it is usually evident to family members or co-workers.

Our diurnal rhythms affect our resilience: onset of toothache is most common in the early morning, osteoarthritic pain in the knee is greatest in the evening and the most intense episodes of angina occur between 2 a.m. and 6 a.m.

During the day we are apertic and the activity uses resources. Our physiology is also exercised in digesting and metabolizing the food we eat. It is not surprising that growth through cell replacement, another necessary function, is most active during the night when there is less metabolic activity, when resources have been freed for the vital renewing process.

There is a physiological price to pay if endogenous cycles are persistently dislocated. When rhythms of sleep and wakefulness are constantly disrupted, physical and cognitive functions deteriorate, leading to ill health.[7]

In short, biological rhythms founded in cellular oscillation can affect our behaviour, and in the reverse position, disordered daily routines and behaviour can disrupt our biological rhythms and physiology.

POTENTIAL AND KINETIC ENERGY

Oscillation can be depicted as a symmetrical, harmonic wave. Springs and pendulums are oscillating objects, their action is reproduced every day by children on a swing in a play area.

There are two forms of energy associated with oscillation, the first, technically kinetic energy, is the energy that we expend pushing the child's swing to start it swinging or oscillating.

---

7   Disruption of the normal circadian clock may promote carcinogenesis. Koukkari and Sothern, *Introducing Biological Rhythms* (Springer Science, 2006) p 487.

The second, technically potential energy, is present in an already oscillating body. It is measured by the force or energy necessary to stop the oscillation. It is evident to anyone who has tried to stop a child's swing that it is often powerful enough to knock an adult over. Our response to events is affected by both potential and kinetic energy.

Unless we are disenchanted with whatever we are doing, whatever we are engaged in has potential energy, a momentum to continue to do it.

We persist in being inactive, or preoccupied with a current interest, until change in our environment attains a sufficient level of kinetic (pushing) energy to overcome the potential (inertia) energy.

In our everyday lives we need to find kinetic energy to respond to a request for help or to be sociable. We often prefer to continue in the potential energy of continuing to read, watch television or enjoy computer games. The potential energy present in the use of a mobile phone is notorious: obstructions go unnoticed, traffic is ignored.

When the degree of change is sufficient, the equivalent of enough kinetic energy to start the child oscillating on the swing, it provokes us to act apertically or recedically. The intensity of kinetic energy that is needed to respond to events is commensurate with the degree of change and of the personal significance that an event has for us.

We are more aroused by our house burning down or by the death of a child than the loss of a wallet or of a pet. We are more aroused by the personal loss of a wallet than the news of a foreign disaster where hundreds have died.

In addition, once we are aroused by change, by an event, the potential energy of response, the momentum of the new apertic or recedic condition, does not dissipate quickly, even if the cause is removed. Agitation can continue after a missing wallet has been found. More serious events take days or weeks to return to equanimity.

It has already been noted that we are fortunate when a night's sleep with REM, dreaming, degrades the potential energy, diminishing the significance of events.

A persistent potential energy becomes attached to our convictions. Once we have arrived at a settled decision about the nature of a physical or social environment – the character of another race of people, a football team, an author, a brand of crisps – the potential energy diminishes any possibility that we will change our mind. It gradually becomes an ingrained or biased attitude.

More constructively, potential energy is associated with the commitments we make in life. If we have made a willing commitment to work or a task, to a relationship, to a religious belief, to a sport, to a field of study, it has potential energy that carries us forward in that specific field.

Overcoming potential energy is often easier for routine events than an unworn path. It is capably managed in professional athletes who 'warm up', stimulating kinetic energy in preparation for a race before the start. It is much more difficult for authors to overcome 'writers' block' ennui.

Possibly the most regrettable consequences of potential energy are evident in corporate behaviour, which has the same characteristics as individual human behaviour. Large organizations have potential energy through opinionated confidence in their own perfection. They receive many criticisms; most are easily dismissed, but the accusations of a 'whistle-blower' within the company who shows that the organization is dysfunctional, or acted illegally, needs a reaction. On many such occasions the organization's potential energy against change will obliterate the intrusion, removing the whistle-blower in one way or another.

Unfortunately for the organization, but fortunately for a free society, the error arises again if they take further questionable steps to suppress the existence of mismanagement, with selected evidence. Each such step makes the final consequence worse. In the UK, for example, the Post Office has recently had to admit to treating many postmasters malignantly, seriously harming their lives.

Potential energy diminishes sensitivity to events. In doing so, it significantly diminishes work for the decision-making facility.

SYNCHRONY AND RELATIONSHIPS

The phenomenon of synchrony reproduces the resonance that occurs in heterogenous objects: windows, for example, rattle harmonically with the throb of a plane flying overhead.

Synchrony of oscillation with 'another', as in a Newton's pendulum, brings a more resilient rhythm. Two cells in synchronous oscillation are similarly reinforced, united in maintaining the rhythm of oscillation, a vital contribution to cellular physiology: synchronicity between two adjacent cells, reinforces the physiology of both cells. It is paralleled in choirs, where the cardiac rhythms of those who are singing can coincide.

Two forms of synchrony are possible between oscillating objects:

i) When two or more 'bobs' oscillate together they have greater potential energy (labelled in this work parallel synchrony).
ii) Two identical but opposite oscillations where the zenith waves of one oscillation coincide with the nadirs of the other (labelled in this work reciprocal synchrony). In reciprocal synchrony, the waves of one precisely mirror the other and can be likened to jigsaw pieces fitting closely together. Electronically, the oscillating waves cancel each other out with the release of energy.

There is no apparent research of reciprocal synchrony in organic fields and little evidence of it in physics. One experiment appears to combine mirrored acoustic waves which produce enough energy to levitate tungsten balls into the air.[8]

Dancing is a fascinating human example of parallel and reciprocal enhancement. In inline country dancing, there is a reinforcing, parallel synchrony between individuals. In ballroom dancing, such as a waltz, the partners mirror each other's movements. As one flexes

---

[8]   Brandt, E. H., 'Acoustic Physics: Suspended by Sound', *Nature* volume 413, 2001, pp 474–475.

a leg forward the other extends the opposing leg backwards, the couple becoming one oscillating body. Both parallel and reciprocal synchrony reinforce each oscillation and can induce a benign, enjoyable emotion.

THE SECOND ERA OF BEHAVIOURAL EVOLUTION

Multicellular Life

The synchrony of parallel oscillation between two cells facilitated the transition from unicellular to multicellular forms of life. Synchrony in reciprocal oscillation resulted in sexual reproduction.

As life on this planet became more temperate the need to repeatedly separate from the environment in sporulation diminished and in one or several species, periodic 'reflex' separation (p 8) was modulated (3 billion years after unicellular life first arose).

The degraded behaviours allowed unicellular life of the same species to congregate in contact and remain in synchrony with each other indefinitely. The assembly of cells can be compared to all coordinated groups where the whole is more than the sum of the individual parts. The advantages that the change provided generated the rapid evolution of multicellular life.

Multicellular-Like Behaviour Through Synchrony Between Individuals

Being in parallel synchrony with others becomes a compulsive behaviour, almost but not quite as powerful as more elemental behaviours. Synchrony or bonding can be displaced by extreme events when there is reversion to individualistic, unicellular-like responses.

Adverse events (p 11) such as fire and extreme benign events such as winning the lottery often propel, even the members of a family, into separating from each other.

Otherwise, parallel synchrony encourages communal living in herds, tribes, flocks, shoals, etc., which brings considerable advantages for the individual and the species.

The drive to be synchronous between two individuals in our society is often self-evident when it occurs. It becomes the object of amusement to others when couples are first 'in love' and delight in finding themselves of one mind about 'everything'.

A sense of synchrony, of both having the same perception of the environment and response to it, first occurs between mother and child. It becomes most compelling and addictive between partners 'in love'. The phenomena are often referred to as 'bonding'. When the opportunity to experience being in synchrony is lost, as in widowhood, our resilience and our ability to maintain good health is diminished.

Japanese cranes, for example, display an unusual degree of synchrony and satisfaction with it, through prolonged rhythmical dancing together at the beginning of courtship. They usually remain with their partner for life and are assiduous parents.

SEXUAL REPRODUCTION

Bonding, or technically the parallel synchrony of 'love', of friendship, of parenting children, plays a significant part in human lives. But reciprocal synchrony is a crucial contribution to sexual reproduction.

The earliest and simplest form of reproduction is parthenogenesis, a process that splits a cell into halves, becoming two cells. The origin of sexual reproduction is actively debated by academic scientists. In this concept it is advanced that two cells (technically gametes) could only associate close together with synchronous oscillations, either parallel or reciprocal. In reciprocal oscillation, like the waltzing dancers, there is a tendency to fusion, to become one oscillatory body, the jigsaw-like fit predisposes to merging with a resulting release of energy and an exchange of DNA. (This merging event produces an extreme benign illusion in our species.) The new cell (technically a zygote), like the result of enlargement through growth, splits in parthenogenetic-like division to multiple cells.

The academic preoccupation with the genetic processes of sexual reproduction has meant that the significant oscillatory and behavioural aspects of the event are ignored. The process can only begin when two cells 'recognize' that they are the same species, through synchrony of their oscillations.

Recognizing that 'another' is the same (species) as oneself is an elemental behaviour. It has not been researched so far.

In reptile and mammalian intercourse, the process of coitus is orchestrated by complex manipulation of the autonomic nervous system, ANS,[9] using both divisions in rapid alternation, to gain a required effect, particularly in male sexual arousal. During coitus, two events are critical. Masculine arousal, penile engorgement, is initiated by parasympathetic activity. This is surprising as parasympathetic activity is usually associated with recedic withdrawal responses. However, on this occasion the process uses a parasympathetic activity: contracting, closing of circulation of blood vessels that is normally applied to the blood vessels in the skin during cold weather. The mechanism contracts or occludes the blood vessels at the base of the penis, closing off return of the blood to the system, so that it accumulates in the penis. It can be compared to blowing up a balloon and retaining the air within it by tying a 'parasympathetic' knot at its neck to prevent escape of the air. The process is followed by a surge of sympathetic activity (apertic-like stimulation) which initiates orgasm and ejaculation, in effect an example of apertic expansiveness upon the environment, in this case the sexual partner.

Putting the physiological innervation into a behavioural dimension, parasympathetic stimulation, which is usually associated with retreat from the environment, can be reinterpreted as submission to the state of the environment. Sympathetic stimulation is associated with expansiveness or intrusion upon a relevant aspect of the environment – in coitus the other person. It can also be interpreted as an aggressive act.

In romantic fiction the alternated progression is often reproduced, the story starts with the female rejecting and dominating, 'leading the male a dance', whilst the male is the suppliant. (In many species the male must chase the female before there is cooperation in coitus. It usefully ensures that the fittest male is the most likely

---

9   The autonomic nervous system coordinates physiological functions. It has two divisions: the sympathetic and the parasympathetic that were originally believed to ready the subject for fight or for flight. In this concept cells can only transmit two 'instructions' to be apertic or recedic. The sympathetic stimulation accords with apertism, the parasympathetic with recedism. In multicellular life they are often agonistic, the sympathetic raises the blood pressure while the parasympathetic lowers it, but they can operate in tandem to achieve a particular function.

to succeed in fertilization.) In traditional romantic fiction, it is followed by the male becoming the dominant partner with acceptance by the female of that dominance.

It is evident from pornographic material that men can be aroused by the initial female dominance that is found in humiliation and cuckolding scenarios. Others appear to be most aroused by the second stage through images of bondage, of rape and force. The many female readers of the socially unacceptable but very successful novel *Fifty Shades of Grey*,[10] that portrays a dominant male and cooperative female partner, suggests that the fantasy of male domination can occasionally appeal to both sexes.

There is one species in which the process is almost theatrically exhibited and frequently seen on TV nature programmes. Coitus in Komodo dragons is preceded by the female ponderously climbing on top of the male before the roles are reversed to achieve successful copulation. Less well known is the unusual behaviour of one shark species. The female bites the male's tail before allowing coitus to take place. In the praying mantis, coitus continues after the female has bitten off the male's head.

UNTOWARD EFFECTS OF PARALLEL SYNCHRONY

There are two consequences of synchrony or 'infectious behaviours', that can be damaging or destructive.

i)   It is very difficult for two people living closely together to differ in their perceptions. In isolated elderly couples when one suffers a recurrent hallucination, the partner can also begin to experience the hallucination and to act upon it. The mutual delusion is called 'folie a deux' and is easily cured for the second partner affected, by separating the couple.

Living with a personality disordered partner often requires the

---

10   James, E. L., *Fifty Shades of Grey* (Arrow, 2012).

sacrifice of personal perceptions and beliefs to a form of 'folie a deux' if the partnership is to continue.

ii) The increased potential energy of individuals and groups in synchrony with one another is self-evident at festivals and, less happily, in riots and lynching parties.

HIERARCHY

On most occasions, cells adjacent to each other in a small multicellular organism would make the same decision and respond to an event in the same way. However, once thousands of cells were assembled as a multicellular organism it became possible for cells at a distance from each other to experience different pH, temperature, or other environmental conditions. The different experiences will provoke different decisions and physiological responses, including the amplitude of oscillation, a discord that must threaten disintegration.

Just as the first nucleus (p 14) coordinated decision and response in single cells, it became advantageous for one cell or a dedicated group of cells to coordinate the oscillation and physiology and the decision-making and response for every cell in the colony. In short, to assume a hierarchical or dominant role. The coordination was implemented through the early autonomic nervous system.

The organic hierarchy is an inflexible contract between the dominant ANS and 'subject' systems. The ANS guarantees a benign homeostatic environment provided the subject systems accept and fulfil the instructions received from the ANS.

The evolutionary step to multicellular life and the physiological coordination has left many species, including our own, with a hierarchical predisposition. It is an insidious, often compulsive behaviour. We almost automatically place people, events and objects in a two-part hierarchy. Film stars, football players and friends are either awesome or 'past it'. Meals are delicious or mediocre. Plays, books and concerts are fantastic or not worthwhile. The second best is little regarded.

When an individual holds an unusually elevated position there is a race to duplicate their appearance, to identify with the 'star', and often a compulsion to associate with those who are regarded as hierarchically higher. Some dream of having tea with the Queen, and football clubs make large profits by selling shirts with the number and name of the team's most successful players to their fans.

Hierarchy permeates and distorts our communication. When we think that an item of information is important, we emphasize it and give it a more loaded significance as we relate it to others. Newspaper editors impose a hierarchy of significance through the size of headlines that they attach to articles and reports.

Manufacturers use the authoritarian power of labels to promote their products.[11] It replicates the placebo success associated with the assurance given to the patient by white-coated authoritarian doctors that the prescribed treatment will bring relief.

Mediaeval societies also knew of the curative power of a hierarchical association; hundreds sought the king's touch to cure their ailments.[12]

As with the pecking order in chickens, individuals can have a higher and a lower position simultaneously. A driver is hierarchically in charge of a car but, if he is wise, he will submit to the traffic lights. Being dominated is more easily accepted if there is another to dominate. On a farm, the sheepdog responds to the minimal signal of a shepherd's whistle but enjoys controlling the herd of sheep. A pernicious hierarchy may occur in prisons where change of environment and motility are circumscribed. Those with the greatest mobility and freedom, the nomads of the steppes, actively reject hierarchy.

In many successful marriages and partnerships, an alternating balance is achieved, with one partner making decisions in one area of

---

[11]   In an experiment by Professor Lesley Regan, reported on 23 April 2009 on BBC2, she demonstrated that branded painkillers brought more relief than identical generic products. (In effect, the brand names carried a visible authority that the medication would diminish the subject's pain.)

[12]   https://history.rcplondon.ac.uk/blog/touching-kings-evil-short-history

the couple's lives whilst the other directs elsewhere. However, many women, and some men, suffer from 'control freaks', from partners who have little authority elsewhere and are addicted to hierarchical dominance at home.

The healthy hierarchical position is being in control of one's life, having the freedom to go where we wish and to choose a pattern of life that we are at ease with. However, the social environment is impaired for everyone when an individual who is addicted to perceiving themselves as 'superior' constantly seeks to demonstrate to him or herself that he, or she, is entitled to dominate events. In that self-deception, city drivers of four-wheel-drive vehicles are four times more likely than drivers of other cars to use hand-held mobile phones and they are less likely to comply with the law on seat belts.[13] Accepting a hierarchy may be life-saving or disastrous: health, for example, can be restored by submitting to medical advice, but total submission to dictators was catastrophic for Europe in the 20th century.

A balanced hierarchical condition is beneficial; unrelieved abasement can cause depression, and it is easy to see that high political status and recognition as a celebrity both become addictive, i.e. have excess momentum or potential energy attached to retaining the elevated position. 'Absolute power corrupts absolutely', Lord Acton, 1887.

Professor Makiko Yamada and colleagues at the National Institute of Radiological Sciences labelled the susceptibility of an individual to believe that they are above others a 'superiority illusion' and found that it was associated with high levels of dopamine in the brain.[14]

Alternatively, the acceptance of hierarchical direction can be attractive because it relieves decision-making, ultimately reducing the need to choose which response attitude to take, to be apertic or recedic.

---

[13]   Walker, Lesley, et al., 'Unsafe driving behaviour and four-wheel drive vehicles: observational study', *BMJ*, Vol 333, 8 July 2006, pp 71–74.

[14]   Yamada M., et al., 'Superiority illusion arises from resting state brain networks modulated by dopamine'. Proceedings of the National Academy of Sciences of the United States of America, 12 Mar. 2013, 110(11):4363-4367.doi:10.1073/pnas.1221681110

Hierarchy is an attribute that often takes precedence over other motivations. Some, possibly most of us, are preoccupied with measuring and comparing our social status in one or another interest, including the model and brand of car we own, our level of education, degree of philanthropy and, for the aged, the status of their grandchildren, or the number of pills they need to consume to keep alive.

There can be ongoing internalized conflict between accepting a socially, politically or family imposed hierarchical position and a desire to be more independent, to be able to make personal decisions. The desire grows in adverse circumstances. It gives rise to disorder and rebellion, a threat to every governing political party. The possibility of disorder usually ensures that ruling political parties maintain as benign an environment as possible for their electorate.

BIAS

The assessment of change in the environment and decision-making consumes resources. Both can be reduced by biased behaviour. For example, if the environment is consistently experienced as adverse, changing conditions do not require a response – require kinetic energy – unless a new event is so substantial that it takes the individual out of default pessimism. The biased behaviour is economic of resources.

It is not possible to identify when the bias characteristic first evolved but it created two existential patterns:

a) A tendency to be recedic or withdrawing, but dependent upon regular fluctuation of the environment for the necessary stimulus of change.

b) Apertically (or optimistically) going out into the environment, moving actively in pursuit of change and the benign.

Both behaviours diminish the significance of events and demand on the decision-making facility.

Biased recedic characters by filtering out the less significant.

Biased apertic characters by inflation, by multiplicity, where the significance of an event is devalued by the number that are experienced.

Barnacles, for example, move little and allow the twice-daily tides to bring change and nutrition. Crab species, their very distant relatives, are more adventurous, actively searching for prey. They are easily caught in cages that, in their unconsidered apertism, they scramble into.

Bias persists into our species with two disparate personality types: one, the recedic, tending towards maintaining the status quo, the other, the apertic, with an underlying tendency to move out, to move on, in one form or another. The dichotomy presages the unending left/right political schism.

We gravitate between (i) looking for invigorating change and unicellular-like independence that prevails in adolescence and young adulthood and (ii) seeking a stable, protected environment, a multicellular-like existence, particularly in old age.

Comment

Bias can take precedence over other behavioural traits, both in its expression and in observation of it by others. Observers become very aware of a subject's predisposition both in animal and human life. A sloth is unthreatening whilst feline species arouse wariness. An elderly fellow pedestrian is overtaken without a thought; an inebriated teenager is avoided if possible.

When we need to suppress bias, suppress our habits of apertic/recedic response, we can feel vulnerable, but new occasions can make it wise to drop our usual dispositions. It occurs when we find ourselves in new environments and we are particularly keen to avoid making a gaffe or making the wrong move.

The occasions arise in unfamiliar circumstances, typically whilst eating for the first time in another society; not knowing whether it is polite to clear one's plate or leave some food on it. (In some societies the plate will be replenished until some food is left upon it.) Not knowing whether it is acceptable to eat from a communal dish with both hands. (A ghastly mistake in societies where the left hand is reserved for cleaning oneself after defecation.) A common uncertainty is about which piece of cutlery to use at a formal dinner.

Visiting a prospective partner's home, and particularly in meeting a partner's parents for the first time, epitomizes the difficulty associated with such events. Being recedically biased is usually believed to be the safest attitude but it can be mistaken for a hostile act, labelled elsewhere as 'passive aggressiveness' – an unfortunate interpretation when the intended attitude is that of recedic submission to the new 'tribe'.

The fear of making a gaffe, the discomforting sense of vulnerability, or a reluctance to deny one's bias, which is commonly asserted to be just plain speaking, can (like agoraphobia) prevent those reluctant to be exposed to unfamiliar social situations from leaving their accustomed environment.

THE FAMILIAR

The basic behavioural need is to define the character of new events, to define whether the environment has changed to being benign or adverse. No occasion is without risk of mishap, it is dangerous to assume that a well-known local environment is totally benign. We need to be aware of adverse circumstances, to know 'where not to go'. To know, for example, where there is a loose aggressive dog, to know which pub is cliquey, to know which restaurant is unhygienic. After adverse circumstances are established, it is safer to go out into the environment.

There is an inherent need to define, to allocate, some aspects of the environment as adverse. The 'other side of the coin' is that whatever is the most familiar is the most benign for us, we know where we stand with it, it provides a secure foundation.

The consequence of current philosophies is that many feel forced to be recedic to 'political correctness', to be 'woke'. They are required to surrender, revoke, deny what has been the hospitable familiar, to feel ashamed of and to reverse what was often a very mild aversion to the unfamiliar into attachment, to put the newly labelled benign on a pedestal and wear sackcloth for their past life. It cannot be surprising that it provokes agonistic reactions that precipitate destructive acts and burgeoning malignant communications online.

In addition, it is possible that committing 'mischief', destabilizing others, is a universal attribute. Such actions can range from critically commenting on one person to a third party and knowing it will be passed on, to practical jokes, to anonymous communications, to the extreme 'mischief' of serial killers and dictators going to war.

A need to be mischievous, to be offensively destructive on occasion, is a unicellular-type rebellion, a need to exercise the alternative to compelling synchrony. I have already posited that there is an alternative to every behaviour that 'strives' to be expressed from time to time. However unconscious, denied or suppressed the behaviour may be, it erupts in one form or another but fortunately can find release in night-time dreaming and, less comfortably, in intrusive thoughts. Intrusive thoughts are now clinically recognized. Possibly, for the first time, individuals are now able to admit to having sociopathic-like fantasies, to having occasional transient thoughts of being violently destructive in relationships, without self-condemnation but can be reassured that the behaviour is in 'the normal range'.

PRECEDENTS OF THE THIRD ERA

In the early second era of behavioural evolution, animal life interacted with other species, developing strategies, motor and sensory skills and different physical forms that enhanced individual survival in the competition for prey and in avoidance of predators.

In the late second era, complex behaviours evolved in mammalian communities that encouraged integration. Living as an integrated group is more successful in foraging and in the detection of predators than it is for a solitary individual.

Integration can only be achieved through synchrony with other members, synchrony is achieved by the ability to 'read the feelings' of other members of the tribe, gaining their acceptance, and in diverting hostility into grooming. These are attributes that can be grouped together as emotional intelligence.

INTELLIGENCE

EMOTIONAL INTELLIGENCE

Both IQ, or problem-solving intelligence, and emotional intelligence enhance the ability of the individual, the group, and the species to survive and are consequently selectively increased through generations.

Knowing others, reading their involuntary emotional responses, can be compared to tracking the clues left by potential prey that disclose where it has been, the direction in which it is heading and its vitality. But the equally valuable ability is knowing oneself, knowing where one is starting from.

KNOWING ONESELF

Monitoring one's own emotions, the ability to know oneself is behavioural 'proprioception'. It is configured from physical proprioception (an unconscious facility) as a framework to build upon.

Extract from an earlier volume: *A New Perception.*[15]

'The physical proprioceptive[16] sub-system is a vital part of

---

15   IBSN (Paperback): 978-1-912892-40-2 Bugler, Robert ,2019.
16   Wikipedia: 'Proprioception, is the sense of the relative position of neighbouring parts of the body and strength of effort being employed in movement. ... It is distinguished from exteroception, by which one perceives the outside

the neuro-muscular system that unconsciously monitors and adjusts muscles and joints to preserve our upright posture. It enables the brain to "know" the position we are in at any time, the point that any new activity commences from. If I want a drink and am lying down, I need to undertake quite different movements to those that I would carry out if I was already sitting. Awareness (largely subconscious) of what direction is up and what is down in the environment and my starting point are critical to undertaking any task. The resource has its own cerebral organ, the cerebellar lobes. The information and myriad slight adjustments are facilitated through its own tracts, which have some of the fastest transmission rates of the nervous system.'

It has recently been recorded (Wikipedia) that, 'The cerebellum is involved in adjusting activities to meet new conditions and research suggests it has a role in the expression of behaviour that is not yet elucidated.' In other words, new research would appear to confirm that the cerebellar system facilitates behavioural as well as physical proprioception.

The physical proprioceptive system is exercised early in life as babies learn how to hold and pass an object from one hand to another. Behavioural proprioception is more gradually established from experiences throughout childhood and early adulthood.

Talented authors can recognize the dynamic of a behavioural phenomenon when others fail to do so. John Bew in his biography of Clement Attlee[17] writes: 'What distinguished him from the pack was not ambition, though he was not without this – so much as a self-awareness lacking in many of his peers.'

---

world, and interoception, by which one perceives pain, hunger, etc., and the movement of internal organs. The brain integrates information from proprioception and from the vestibular system into its overall sense of body position, movement, and acceleration.'

[17]   Bew, John, *Citizen Clem: A Biography of Attlee* (Riverrun, 2017) p 200.

The crucial sense is being aware of which behavioural mode, apertic or recedic, we are in. Whether we are likely to respond to a situation in an asserting mode or in gauging and assessing the circumstances.

The skill can be compared to a chess player who knows without thinking about it that he/she is behaving most sensibly in a recedic mode to safeguard the king or in the alternative, being apertic, to checkmate an opponent.

Physical proprioception has little consciousness, and behavioural proprioception has even less, so it is easily ignored when we are distracted by external events, particularly when we are sexually attracted. Unfortunately, just when we need to be aware of being over apertic, possibly too intrusive, we can fail to do so, or do not want to recognize it. Without behavioural proprioception we can behave badly. For many, it needs to be better cultivated.

KNOWING OTHERS

The other pillar of emotional intelligence is knowing others, being able to 'read' another's emotional responses.

Some individuals, such as successful poker players, manage to conceal their response to events. Children who have been treated cruelly, and suffered more when they have shown emotion, also learn to suppress it. Psychopaths learn to flag up emotions they do not actually feel. Actors find it possible to display a false emotion by conceiving a personality and an appropriate event. Different races vary in the quality and degree of emotional response that individuals display or consider to be socially acceptable.

Those circumstances apart and unlike emotions conveyed by verbal language, the involuntary phenomena are usually honest revelations of how an individual feels and they can be difficult to suppress.

Human emotions are disclosed in facial expressions, facial colour, posture or body language, timbre of voice and an olfactory component that may not be consciously registered.

a) Facial expression. We have many small facial muscles that show fine degrees of emotion. Combinations of eyes, eyebrows, lips, nose and cheek movements declare both the different nature and degree of response.

b) Facial colour. The flush through vascular dilatation in anger and the pallor through vascular contraction in shock are easily recognised, and we are, almost unconsciously, aware of much finer differences of emotion in conversations.

From *The Times* (20 March 2018):

'We are used to the idea that skin colouration can convey extreme emotion, but a recent study has shown that it is an effective signal of all the moods in between too. Most people think they can spot what others are feeling by looking at their facial muscles, but it turns out that we can do almost as well just by looking at their cheeks. The research was carried out by Alex Martinez, from the Ohio State University [...] For his study, published in the journal *Proceedings of the National Academy of Sciences*, he wanted to see if these blood vessels served a purpose by "signalling" emotion. He and his colleagues trained a computer to spot subtle differences of colour in faces expressing different emotions. ... More than 80 per cent of the time people were able to identify the one that matched the emotion ... He said that this showed just how crucial picking up on subtle social cues must be for humans.'

This is crucial for successful integration in whatever group we are part of.

c) Body postures. Both sitting and standing postures indicate emotions. A person sitting to the back of a chair, leaning forward, with their head nodding along with the discussion implies that they are open, relaxed and generally ready to listen, recedic, receptive. Otherwise, a listener who has their legs and arms crossed, perhaps with a foot kicking slightly, implies that they are feeling impatient, apertic and emotionally detached from the discussion.

d) Timbre of voice. This is perhaps the easiest to imitate so actors use it frequently to try to convey emotion.

e) Possibly an olfactory element. It may be a myth, but some victims are reported to smell of fear.

Registering one's own and another's emotions are vital attributes. It is particularly important to recognize when there is dichotomy in their expression.

Our physiology and our emotional 'functions' are based upon finding and responding to the material and social environment as adverse or benign. We are predisposed to define new events as one or the other. We feel ill at ease when events have conflicting characteristics. The discomfort will be greatest when facial and body language differ in anyone we are engaged with. If they advertise synchrony but their expression suggests disregard, it is unwise to depend upon their goodwill. A lack of wrinkles around the eyes suggests a fake or sham smile.

Television editors focus upon actions that indicate difference with what is being said and direct the camera to an interviewee's clutched fingers or feet tapping away. Honest emotions, visible to others, are essential to trust and cooperation.

Our ability to define the environment accurately is essential to our self-confidence and self-esteem. We think less of ourselves when we find we have believed a lie. Dishonesty is so disliked that perjury has been made a serious crime. We are discomfited when we find that a relative or an acquaintance we thought we knew well had associations or beliefs that were never communicated, or that we were never made aware of.

Ability to recognize involuntary emotional signals in others cannot be learnt in hours or days. Some individuals appear to have a 'natural' aptitude, but for most of us it is only through childhood years of living in a community that most of us acquire the necessary skills.

In acquiring speech and language, we can convey our own emotions and ask how others are feeling. It can be an honest exchange or a misleading one; it lacks the purity of involuntary display. When an acquaintance vocalizes with gestures the emotion that they wish to display, they are projecting it forcefully. Like a magician's sleight of hand, it diminishes our sensitivity to involuntary display and it can hide dishonesty in the emotion that is being vocalized.

Children may not follow a conversation between adults but often have unknowing awareness of the real feelings of those participating in the conversation, sensing more accurately than their parents whether another adult's friendship is sincere or not.

PRIMATE INTELLIGENCE

The evolution from unicellular to multicellular life was facilitated by change to a more equable climate, it diminished the need to make rapid, polarized decisions and responses.

The effect of the change can be compared to a different set of traffic lights. When the lights are limited to short red/green intervals, pedestrians must be alert and immediately respond to the changing lights. When an amber interval is introduced, they no longer need to rush, they can continue to talk to companions as they cross over.

In relaxed, temperate conditions, single cells can behave like the pedestrians talking to each other whilst crossing. They can remain in contact together and move into a synchronous multicellular existence.

Moving forward to just six million years ago, the East African climate fluctuated between dry periods and temperate intervals. Vegetation flourished in the temperate periods and created a reliably benign environment with less polarization between foraging and guarding. It had surprising consequences.

FOUNDATION OF INTELLIGENCE

When polarization and response are relaxed it is possible for both benign and adverse aspects to be absorbed, to register both almost simultaneously. It increases the volume of information available for the decision-making process.

The advantage can be illustrated in a personal, theatre-like, representation. I find on starting to return to my home from a London terminus that there are two trains advertised from different platforms: a slow train (adverse) stopping at several stations that is cheap to travel on. There is a fast train (benign) on another platform that is leaving shortly. It is more expensive but significantly reduces the journey time.

In a recedic mood, I choose the slow, cheaper train; in an apertic mood, I pay more and choose the fast train as I would like to arrive home as early as possible.

However, if both trains can be accessed from either side of one platform, I am able to see advantages and disadvantages that I might otherwise have missed, such as a friend I want to meet getting onto one train or that passengers are already standing on the train I was about to board whilst the other has unoccupied seats. It is only by accessing change in the environment, from the one platform, holding both points of view, that I can make the most advantageous choice.

In the most primitive circumstances, change in the environment had to have a benign or adverse quality for it to be registered. The system ensured rapid, life-saving responses. During evolution, the need to make immediate decisions gradually diminished. In effect, benign and adverse qualities lost intensity and gradually reached a point where the individual details of an event could be registered with minimal or no differentiation. It allowed multiple details to be held in consciousness simultaneously. The more details that are available, the more intelligent a decision can be made.

MEMORY – FILING

Acquiring more information by absorbing adverse and benign aspects of an event is a half-step to greater intelligence, the other half is retaining or storing the information. We remember the unusual, the more emotionally arousing experiences, and those that have intruded on our own lives more than others. Unfortunately, neither is of much assistance in acquiring the necessary knowledge, vocabulary, ability to read, ability to add, subtract, multiply and divide, to function in modern urban society. The necessary knowledge is available in most societies but retaining it so that it can be subsequently applied to solve problems is more difficult.

Revision, repeatedly absorbing the information, has been the traditional method of retaining it. The easiest way to acquire information, remember and apply it is through copying others in an integrated, related group.

The Times (25 January 2022) reported that in two chimpanzee troops, or tribes, living within 4 miles of each other, one had learnt how to use stones to crack nuts, the other tribe had not acquired the skill and still failed to do so when they were provided with examples and opportunity to learn. Professor Koops concluded that the knowledge was acquired by being passed on through generations, possibly initiated by one particularly intelligent member. She notes that 'crucial social skills are necessary for a cumulative culture'.[18]

In a contrast, *The Times* (17 February 2022) reported research on magpies in Australia. The article focused on the difficulty of ensuring that tracking devices remained in place on the magpies. Unlike the failure of the chimpanzees to acquire knowledge, the magpies, with much smaller brains than chimpanzees, discovered how to detach the devices from each other and showed others how to do it.[19]

---

[18]   Professor Kathelijne Koops, University of Zurich, published in *Human Nature Behaviour*, January 2022.
[19]   Australian magpies *Gymnorhina tibicen* cooperate to remove tracking devices.

The difference is that heterogenous human-chimpanzee asso-ciation lacked the necessary synchronicity, hinted at in Professor Koops, the magpies were taught by copying others of the 'same flock', often close family.

Intelligence:

i) is derived from the ability to absorb benign and adverse elements of change of the environment at the same time.

ii) The ability to store and retrieve information or knowledge is as important as the ability to absorb detail.

iii) Children incorporate information copied in the family more successfully than information received from other sources.

Crampton, Joel, Frere, Celine H. and Potvin, Dominique A.: 'Notably, removal was observed to involve one bird snapping another bird's harness at the only weak point, such that the tracker was released. This behaviour demonstrates both cooperation and a moderate level of problem solving, providing potential further evidence of the cognitive abilities of this species.'

IDENTITY

Identity is a sense of self that has emotion attached to it, pleasure in feeling self-esteem or discomfort in experiencing loss of credibility or shame. Recognition of it as a behavioural attribute originated in the mid-19th century and began with an accident to Phineas Gage, a railroad worker. His personality changed dramatically after his left cerebral frontal lobe was severely damaged by a penetrating iron rod in 1848. Previously a well-balanced, motivated individual, he became bad-tempered and uncaring. Simplistically, he lost respect for himself and how he behaved.

Identity has multiple labels. Sigmund Freud's 'ego' is perhaps best known. It is also known as psyche, Ka, Ba, self-esteem and personality.

Identity, in this concept, is the form in which others 'see' us and we 'see' ourselves, our character or personality.

Like our physical self, identity grows through childhood to maturity. Self-esteem should be nurtured but not excessively encouraged by parents and others who care for children. The metamorphosis of identity after puberty is as radical as the physical changes. It can be compared to the release of insect pupae from a carapace or passing out of the prison gate without direction, not knowing which way to go or what is possible. It brings both a flood of choices and a demand for decisions.

ANTECEDENTS OF IDENTITY

Technically the frontal lobe 'is responsible (in a managing sense) for higher cognitive functions such as memory, emotions, impulse control, problem solving, social interaction, and motor function. Damage to the neurons or tissue of the frontal lobe can lead to personality changes, difficulty in concentrating or planning, and impulsivity.'[20]

It is also posited that the frontal lobes hold a 'motor homunculus' within their function. It is a framework or holographic-like image of ourselves, an image with which we can give ourselves self-esteem from the way we imagine we look, in being well groomed, or feel ashamed if we believe we have an unkempt appearance. The self-image of other species will be their smell (skunks) or their sound (many birds), the instruments of their expansion rather than their physical appearance. Predators expand upon the environment through claws and teeth; when they lose those instruments, they lose their presence. The image we have of ourselves, our identity, is the instrument of our presence. When it is well grounded in reality, others will have the same image.

Recent work suggests that the frontal lobes, which show development until the mid-thirties, make decisions. In this concept, decisions are made in the hind brain, the frontal lobes influence the decisions of the hind brain to reinforce self-identity or protect it.

The gradual increase in the size of the human brain has occurred through multiplication of axons that carry impulses from one site to another.

'These comparative analyses indicate that the evolutionary process of neocorticalization in primates is mainly due to the progressive expansion of the axonal mass that implement global communication, rather than to the increase in the number of

[20] https://www.healthline.com/human-body-maps/frontal-lobe.
Accessed 21 November 2021

cortical neurons and the importance of high neural connectivity in the evolution of brain size in anthropoid primates.'[21]

Increase of connectivity must facilitate the influence of frontal lobe (identity) on the hind brain executing decisions.

*　*　*

We are not descended from one or other of the Great Ape species but arose from a common ancestor. Our evolution from that ancestor has not so far left evidence of its nature but it is reasonable to assume that the earliest hominid communities had similarities to chimpanzee and bonobo communal existence that we can observe today and detect the early behaviours that eventually generated and expanded to modern-day human identity and its pervasive influence on everything we do.

The essential need for all the members of the bonobo community is to integrate with the complex relationship and communication behaviours of the troop. The most important skill for the young to acquire is acceptance by the community, in this concept, emotional intelligence or how to appease and engage successfully. It can only be acquired by observing how others achieve it and how they can gain respect.

The individuals who build the best nests and find the ripest fruit are copied. 'Imitation being the sincerest form of flattery.' Respect is also given to elderly females who settle disputes and restore harmony. But some members of chimpanzee communities find satisfaction in 'asocial' behaviour, for example, in concealing the discovery of ripe fruit, in cheating and deceiving others.

One well-recorded behaviour, which has no obvious survival advantage and perplexes observers, is that of dominant males beating their chests. In the context of this work, the alpha male is

---

[21]   Hofman,Michel A., 'Evolution of the human brain: when bigger is better', Netherlands Institute for Neuroscience, Royal Netherlands Academy of Arts and Sciences, Amsterdam, Netherlands. Front. Neuroanat., 27 March 2014, https://doi.org/10.3389/fnana.2014.00015

saying, 'This is me, this is what I am.' The behaviour underlines an unrecognized but fundamental element of communication. When I make a statement, 'The weather has turned worse', the first and most relevant person I am making that statement to is myself. I am reinforcing my perception of what the reality is. The phenomenon is used in psychoanalytical analysis. The analyst would register the gorilla's need for reassurance of self-value – and wonder why it was necessary.

Behaviour that can be interpreted as 'reinforcing identity' has been reported by chimpanzee keepers in zoos. Chimpanzees have been observed engaging in risky behaviour for no obvious gain. And young chimpanzees sometimes spend time screwing up their faces in various expressions, possibly practising deception.

In effect, chimpanzees begin to show a desire for self-esteem or identity and for finding ways to acquire it.

HUMAN IDENTITY

As we approach adulthood, the first choice thrust upon us is the field in which to work, compete or find enjoyment: sport, academic, profession, business or opting out in hedonism. Whatever inherent skills we have may contribute to our choice, but others around us are very influential. The achievements of other members of our peer group can be a factor, and parental pressure can either persuade us to follow their choice or provoke rebellion and a rejection of their mores and lifestyle.

When we have found a field we can commit to, we categorize our self-identity in relation to that field. The number of books the author sells, the number of people who vote for an MP, the choice and value of shares purchased.

Identity often becomes attached to physical appearance or reinforcement by material possessions: the size of car, of house, the value of jewellery. A hierarchical position in society is much sought after and rewarded with desirable prizes: knighthoods, Oscars and

Olympic gold medals. The reward, like amassing a fortune, is seldom sufficient, as the desire to reinforce self-identity parallels drug addiction. Like any addiction, it can only be transiently satisfied.

Identity varies in intensity from one individual to another. It is not susceptible of measurement or scientific manipulation except through artificially conceived and defined aspects: pride, degree of narcissism, of paranoia. There is no calibration of identity as a 'whole', the degree that it is present in any one of us, or of its sensitivity to events.

The need to secure our identity is most evident when we seek to protect it from being harmed and otherwise in our efforts to reinforce it.

In protection, we compulsively distance ourselves from adverse events that range from minor mishaps to major disasters. When things go wrong we deny as automatically as an involuntary reflex that we have had any part in the reverse. The reaction was encapsulated by President Kennedy after the disastrous 'Bay of Pigs' invasion of Cuba. He told a journalist, 'Victory has a hundred fathers, defeat is an orphan.'

In other circumstances, we enhance our identity by spontaneously joining in with any successful endeavours that arise. We give ourselves 'positive strokes' when we tell others about events in which we have played an active part. There is also satisfaction in voicing 'negative strokes', in disparaging, ridiculing the success of others. Tabloid newspapers offer a daily selection of negative strokes, as they trawl through the failings of celebrities whom they have previously idolized.

There is one avenue to choose an identity for ourselves: our names. Few feel that the birth names they were given reflect the identity they wish to be. Adolescents often modify their names or create new ones.

When we are weak with physical illness, we become recedic, withdrawing from the environment, from exchange with other people. When our identity feels vulnerable, when we are not coping well with our responsibilities or the expectations of others, we have a fragile identity and can interpret any comment or question as a criticism. We respond aggressively to protect ourselves from feeling more diminished.

In as much as we recognize our identity, we blame ourselves for our lack of charisma, lack of worldly success and questionable success in relationships. As a result, it is easy, especially when we are young, to turn to punishing ourselves, inflicting injury on ourselves for the perceived failure, of failure to make the right decisions, and, sometimes, to ultimately commit suicide.

Opportunities to cultivate our identity, our self-esteem, have been displaced throughout the last century. We no longer grow our own vegetables or make our own clothes. Dishwashers, computers and service industries complete the chores we used to undertake for ourselves. George Orwell recorded in *Down and Out in Paris and London* that the lowest-status workers in the hotel kitchen, those who washed the dishes, could find pride in how quickly they could complete the task.[22]

In the absence of opportunity for positive strokes, we falsify them by aligning ourselves with individuals and groups that are flourishing, entertainment celebrities and sports celebrities, often leading football players and their teams in the UK.

In alternate activity, when no satisfying source of positive strokes can be found, fabricating powerful negative strokes by anonymously abusing others on the internet satisfies some individuals, now labelled 'trolls'.

We do not usually beat our chests like alpha male primates but relate how we have disconcerted others by what we have said or how we have behaved and of taking dangerous risks. It is usually interpreted as boasting, showing off, even narcissistic. Quite often, however, the raconteur is not completely confident of the appropriateness or wisdom of their own behaviour. When they relate

---

[22] Orwell, George, *Down and Out in Paris and London*, first published 1933. Available at https://gutenberg.net.au/ebooks01/0100171h.html

the event in company, they put the episode in a 'better context' every time, with the secondary purpose of trawling for reinforcing responses. It can be difficult to avoid giving the raconteur the response that they want, to turn their wish that you are in synchrony with them into refusal. Audiences can find themselves laughing at jokes which, on reflection, are humourless, even malign.

We act cooperatively in giving others mild reinforcement of identity and in eschewing criticism of others. Those who are most skilful in the exercise are described as 'charming'.

We are generally socially responsible in our lives, occasionally slipping into in a selfish mode. There are a few who quietly build identity by dedicating their lives to 'good causes', whilst others with an asocial bias reinforce self-esteem by habitually defrauding the public and other criminal activity.

Gaining, losing and regaining self-identity is the substance of fiction and central to many novels.

Two Paths: Chimpanzees and Hominids

Chimpanzees live in an Eden-like environment, largely at ease with each other. They are able to forage on the ground, in the tree canopy and in forest pools, and as a troop they have a multiple awareness to detect and avoid predators. Existence is unchallenging, there is no equal in ability and agility – except their own kind. Consequently, it is not surprising that from time to time they look for challenge in warfare with their own species and cannibalism.[23] Feasting on an opponent is particularly satisfying as it removes all evidence that the opponent ever existed.

Once individual chimpanzees achieved integration, the Eden-like existence removed any need to learn how to socialize and how to forage because the behaviour of other members of the troop could

---

[23]   Bygott, J. D., 'Cannibalism Among Wild Chimpanzees', *Nature* vol 238, 1972, pp 410–411. Abstract: Cannibalism has been observed twice in East African chimpanzee populations. This behaviour is rarely seen among wild mammals and is hitherto unrecorded in non-human primates.

always be copied. The community resource resembles the 21st-century instant access to the internet, it removes the need to learn the emotional intelligence of communicating face to face or how to find one's own way to the supermarket in a new town. Any skill that is not exercised decays. Decay is evident in chimpanzees' poor ability to learn from others, even their own kind. There is academic recognition of the poor facility for learning sociability.[24]

In this concept, modification of two elemental attributes placed hominids on a different path to other primates. The first is a stronger drive to experience change. It encouraged migration, which had the added advantage of moving away from intraspecies warfare and cannibalism. The second augmented trait was hierarchy. Without leadership, without an individual taking responsibility for decision-making, unplanned migration must be a disaster. When hierarchy is in place, higher status is facilitated by intelligence and physical skill, and once acquired, they also reinforce identity. Male status and physical ability appeal to females when choosing who to mate with. It is multiplied by the second stage of coitus. The physiological process, the reciprocal synchrony, amplifies magnetic attraction. In effect, the pursuit of hierarchy and reinforcement of identity potentiate each other and will be propagated by 'female selection of the fittest'.

The hierarchical trait can be seen in our own everyday life as many seek dominance and notoriety. But a more significant aspect of the influence of hierarchy in human life arises from an elemental hierarchical contract.

---

[24] 'This study is new in showing a species difference in readiness to incorporate social information into one's own repertoire,' study researcher Edwin van Leeuwen, a doctoral student at the Max Planck Institute for Psycholinguistics in the Netherlands, told Live Science. ['8 Humanlike Behaviors of Primates']

HIERARCHICAL CONTRACT

A contract-like system was first established between the nucleus and other constituents of the cell. In effect, in the single cell or prokaryote, the nucleus dictates to the other tissues 'if you follow and only if you precisely follow my orchestration, my instructions, I will guarantee you a benign, homeostatic internal environment.'

In multicellular life, the autonomic nervous system duplicates the nucleic role, managing physiology and ensuring reliable homeostasis.

Once a formula has evolved in organic life, the formula is a tool that can be applied in circumstances far removed from the original purpose.

The contract is established in ape species. Young chimpanzees integrate the example provided by adult behaviour and duplicate it, the inset behaviour ensures social acceptance as an adult and avoids fatal exclusion from the tribe.

The hierarchical contract has become integrated in human behaviour without arousing any conscious awareness of its presence. A contract that charges parents to ensure a benign environment and the child to follow the 'instructions', like chimpanzee young, of the parents' behaviour.

The parents' actual behaviour, not how they project themselves, not how they tell the child to behave, but their involuntary emotions, their responses to events and the pattern of their lives, all this material eventually contributes to the child's identity.

When the parent is absent or unavailable, elder siblings and the peer group are influential. In deprived circumstances those who make the environment a little more benign for the child, can also become very influential.

When there is a slight loss of benign circumstances children respond emotionally with tears or grumbling.

When they experience what is, for them, a radical loss, children frequently become anorexic or depressed.

The most damaging consequence arises because the formula (parents are the source of benign care) makes it almost impossible to blame parents for the deterioration of circumstances.

The only alternative to the parents being responsible is to believe that they themselves are at fault. The sense of responsibility has been noted by families, and those who have worked with children for decades. Following a dramatic or tragic event, children will become convinced that they are responsible for the event and show acute distress that is resistant to any attempt by others to ease it. Typical events are parental illness, death of a sibling or father becoming unemployed. Children become convinced that the disaster has occurred because they have failed, they have not been good enough in following or fulfilling 'the instructions'.

The sense of not being good enough is resistant; it persists into adulthood creating a predisposition to depression and a handicapped identity.

It should be self-evident that any disorder will be much greater if it is the parent, or one in loco parentis, who has actually caused the environment to become adverse.

For children in the mid-childhood hierarchical contract period, the parent model makes all the decisions on the benign/adverse quality of events and appropriate responses, they have minimal apparatus of their own for decision-making. For example, when children are asked for their opinion on a television interview, they happily replicate their parents' opinions as their own.

They are usually anxious to avoid any personal responsibility for ephemeral events: 'Please, sir, it wasn't me, sir', whenever possible.

The consequences of abuse, of conscious maltreatment of children, will be returned to later.

Childhood vulnerability is a disadvantage but it is possible that the formula facilitates the ability of our species to acquire and store more information, through education, than other species.

* * *

Before setting out the exigencies of childhood – and parenting – the basic behavioural attributes are summarized below.

OUR COMPOSITE BEHAVIOURAL CONSTITUTION

Our response to change, our behaviour, is shaped by every evolutionary step from the elemental responses to identity:

A BALANCED RECEDISM–APERTISM

Like all organic life we have two basic behaviours: to be open to, to intrude upon and ultimately to exploit the environment or to withdraw from it. We are not as genetically biased as some species to be recedic, to behave like sloths or to be constantly apertically active as rats.

We can be biased as individuals, and physiological disorder can modify the balance. In the very rare Kleine-Levin syndrome,[25] those affected fluctuate between extreme recedic and apertic behaviour. In psychiatric disorder, in depression, there is a lack of kinetic energy, of motivation, whilst overactivity dominates in manic states.

---

[25]   Kleine-Levin syndrome is a rare disorder that primarily affects adolescent males. It is characterized by recurring but reversible periods of excessive sleep (up to 20 hours per day). Affected individuals are completely normal between episodes. It may be weeks or more before symptoms reappear. (Modified extract from National Institute of Neurological Disorders and Stroke site)

NEED TO EXPERIENCE CHANGE

There is wide variation in the drive to experience change, depending on age, inherited characteristics and the state of the physical and social environment. When circumstances are adverse, we are all motivated to move away, to seek change.

We have found ways, or excuses, to gain change in our lives. They range from mediaeval pilgrimages to business conferences. Students travel during gap years and billionaires rocket out to space.

Change can be a vital experience. Occasionally babies have no interest in feeding. Providing change can help. Moving (whilst well covered up) outside to winter frost stimulated one to start feeding whilst another responded to being in a bath with another baby.

NEED TO CONSERVE ENERGY

It is possible that a genetic bias to conservation of energy predisposes to overeating and little exercise. It can be reinforced through childhood experience when relaxed parental attitudes may result in lifetime obesity. As with other traits, the longer it is in place the more installed it becomes and the more difficult to modify.

HOMEOSTASIS

Homeostasis is a contradiction to the need to experience change. The behaviours should not be seen to be in conflict, rather as two 'voices' crying for satisfaction, crying loudest when they have been unsatisfied for a prolonged period. For example, soldiers who have fought in foreign countries for several years, long to return to the homeostatic conditions of their own homes.

OSCILLATORY PHENOMENON

Synchrony predisposes to friendship; asynchrony makes it unlikely. Once both parallel and reciprocal synchrony oscillations occur, sexual attraction can follow.

Oscillations supplement both the recedic and apertic natures of our response to events. They cause a rapid response to some stimuli and a slow response to others, exemplified in a child's differing responses to 'Would you like a sweet?' and 'Time to go to bed'.

Potential energy causes persistent emotional arousal after life-changing events.

SOCIAL MULTICELLULAR AND INDIVIDUAL UNICELLULAR

We enjoy, probably need, both company and solitary intervals; excess of one can predispose us to search for the other.

SEPARATION FROM LETHAL EVENTS

We seek to escape, in fear, from potentially lethal events, or to remove, 'take out', whatever is experienced as a threat, in anger.

HIERARCHY

We have different degrees of awareness of hierarchies in both the social environment and of our own position. Personal hierarchical status is acutely important for the identity of some, of little relevance to others. But for almost everyone, there is sensitivity to hierarchy in one context or another: family, work, creative skills and financial position, size of house, size of car, etc.

BIAS

We can have a susceptibility to bias which can become attached to many aspects such as always seeing the best – or the worst – in others. Showing a preference for male or female authors, is an example.

THE INHERENT PROGRAMME

There is a progression of behavioural maturation through childhood that requires experiences (to be set out later) for the child to acquire a balanced resilient identity.

PARENTING

Inherent human attributes, present at birth, are established during childhood by being enhanced or diminished through the experiences a child receives. This is particularly true of the parenting attribute(s). If a child has had committed parenting, the experience will be reinforced and reproduced later in life with their own progeny.

INTELLIGENCE

We have two forms of intelligence, and their acquisition and growth depend upon genetic factors and the experiences we receive.

MEMORY

Compared to other animal life, we have exceptional memory, especially for events that are accompanied by strong emotion.

DECISION-MAKING RESOURCE

We have one decision-making resource that can be overloaded, predisposing to mental illness (set out later). It is posited that a familial susceptibility to schizophrenia, evident in identical twins, suggests that the fragility of that resource, of resilience to stressful events, is genetically influenced.

COPYING BEHAVIOUR

We can all copy behaviour that appears to be interesting or bring reward. Copying follows on from the involuntary attribute of falling into synchrony with others.

CENTRE OF GRAVITY

Our identity can be compared to the centre of gravity of a body or an object. 'The centre of gravity predicts the behaviour of a moving body when acted upon by gravity.' It can be rewritten as: Identity predicts human behaviour when acted upon by events.

We place ourselves at the centre of events. For example, Church leaders bemoan the effects of paedophile scandals on the Church, before recognizing the injury to the victims.

Celebrities relate common illnesses and mishaps that occur to all of us, as if their suffering is exceptional, even unique.

Lack of a centre of gravity, of identity, of self-esteem is an uncomfortable vacuum assuaged by alcohol, opium and other addictive substances.

* * *

Both for ourselves and other species, behavioural evolution parallels the evolution of complex games. Different evolutionary stages provide a variety of behavioural resources and skills, comparable to the different resources of chess pieces. Whichever resource 'identity' considers is most likely to produce a desired effect is deployed.

As with a game of chess, an unexpected intervention, an event, can change perception of environment and the value and use of all the remaining pieces. We and other mammals such as dogs and cats can see places and people in a different perspective after significantly adverse or benign events.

CHILDHOOD

Ontogenetic influences can be discerned in the behavioural growth of children.

In evolving from unicellular to multicellular forms, survival ceased to depend upon maintaining and protecting cellular physiology and moved to the ability to find prey and avoid predators, to 'survival of the fittest', in competition with other species.

Agility, large size and power are significant advantages in prey/predator survival but in the interval between parturition and achieving an adult condition, progeny are vulnerable.

Multiple strategies evolved; the earliest was the production of large numbers of eggs in the expectation that enough survive to perpetuate the species. It is a successful strategy but wasteful of resources. Some species learnt to use the material environment to provide protection, depositing eggs in inaccessible locations. Containing progeny and nurturing them until they achieve adult form proved to be the most efficient. It was perfected in mammalian life.

During intrauterine growth the human embryo ontogenetically revisits some of the stages of physical evolution, passing, for example, through a phase with fish-like gills. It is possible to track an ontogenetic-like progression that repeats behavioural evolution, after birth and through childhood.

BABIES

Newly born babies move from a sensory deprivation environment to a kaleidoscopic world flooded with visual, auditory and tactile stimuli.

When one sensory experience emerges more powerfully than others, it will either be benign, emotionally pleasant to the baby, or adverse. If it is adverse, the baby has two separation responses, obscuring the adverse change visually with tears and auditorily with loud crying or withdrawing completely in sleep.

The baby is used to an environment, in utero, that provided every necessity without effort and maintained a benign condition, which included the mother's presence. When the baby's environment replicates that state, it is benign. When it fails to do so, or if it becomes internally or externally uncomfortable, it is adverse.

There is a gradual recognition of the parents/carers, especially the mother, of those who prevent or relieve adverse circumstances and a gradual adjustment of the baby's inherent biological rhythms to a diurnal routine.

Usually by six or seven weeks, eye-to-eye contact begins; it is the first parallel synchrony exercise. Eye-to-eye contact declares 'we are of the same species, I want you to enter into synchrony with me, coordinate with my perceptions and responses.'

They are the first steps of moving from the individualistic or unicellular condition to multicellular-like synchrony with others of ones' own kind. The process needs the baby to have the facility be in synchrony (it is not universal) and the carers to cultivate the attribute through physical holding, showing pleasure in doing so, singing softly and moving together in rhythm with the song. It also helps to communicate in a form that the baby can relate to, by alternately echoing, returning, the sounds the baby makes. It is the first rotation of apertic (making the noise) and recedic (listening) positions, the first conversation.

Babies are aware of whether whoever is caring for them is offering synchrony by the way they are held with confidence, by the gentle warmth with which they are talked to or sung to, face to face.

The relationship gradually moves to more purposeful exchange of information. Giving the impression, with enjoyed facial expression and words, that the new experience the baby is going to be introduced to will be benign. In weaning, for example, hopefully the baby will be influenced by the message the person feeding it tries to convey. If that is not successful and the baby finds a new taste unpleasant, both food and the attitude of the person offering food, need to be obstructed with a double volume of noise and tears.

As the baby gets older, becomes an infant, carers begin to expect the infant to fit in with them, to cooperate when being bathed, when being fed. It is easy for the infant to cooperate with simple expectations but the expectations to cooperate should increase. A conflict arises between the baby's residual individualistic unicellular drive to be able to control events and the alternative acceptance that whoever is parenting knows best.

No one likes to give up privileges they have enjoyed, and some infants are desperate to show themselves that they can continue in control, that they can have what they want. It results in the notorious 'terrible twos' temper tantrums, which can be overwhelming to both parties. The internalized infant conflict can begin earlier than the second birthday and occasionally never seems to be capable of resolution.

Most infants gradually discover that a world managed by the adults is more rewarding and secure. However, dreams and fantasies of the world being there solely for them remain and continue throughout life. Boys imagine having controlling guns or other weapons. Girls can imagine being a princess, whose every wish is satisfied.

Adults continue with the fantasy in watching Marvel films or the fantasy of buying winning Euromillion lottery tickets, envisaging having enough money to fulfil any wish.

The infant gradually grows into mid-childhood, a potentially vulnerable period for behavioural development.

MID-CHILDHOOD

Parents have always hoped and largely believed that children are resilient, relatively unaffected by adverse events, and early research tended
to support that assumption. In recent years it has become evident
that children may not show disturbed behaviour at the time that an
adverse event occurs, but the event can have a damaging influence
through creating a susceptibility to personality disorder in adulthood.

SEXUAL ABUSE OF CHILDREN

It was noted above that psychiatry has been influenced by
changing philosophies. They have been relatively minor compared
to the changing attitudes to parenting and care of children, and
notably during the last 70 years, in beliefs relating to the introduction of children to sexuality. They have moved since the 1930s
from telling children nothing to, for some families in late 1960s,
including children in adult sexual activity. Since the 1970s it has
been recognized that using children for sexual arousal is a severely
damaging abuse.

Currently in the UK, sexual instruction is compulsory at age
eleven. Some mature eleven-year-old children will already have the
information; other, uninformed, children can be dismayed to discover
what their parents do in their bedroom. Children differ widely in
their maturity, in their ability to incorporate the information.

Growing awareness of the extent of sexual abuse and its
damaging effects on children, from the late 1970s initiated an active
search for physical and behavioural evidence of abuse. One invented
sign was that of anal sphincter reflex opening on separating a child's
buttocks. Another tested children's acceptance of being touched,
from touching hands to moving towards the genital area. Both led
to innocent parents being mistakenly accused of sexual abuse.

Many who are intelligent and educated find it difficult to understand why 'an early introduction of children to sensuality' is damaging

and hint that the distress of the victims is manufactured for sympathy and compensation. Those who work in the field are well acquainted with how damaging it is to children of all ages but find it puzzling why mid-childhood children, between infancy and early adolescence, are often the most severely affected by the experience.

In this concept, the childhood hierarchical contract (p 52), makes childhood vulnerability to abuse and its damaging effect on self-confidence and self-respect in adulthood a logical consequence.

ADVERSE CHILDHOOD EVENTS (ACE) AND PERSONALITY DISORDER

From the NHS information sites:

> 'Incidence of ACE: In a 2014 UK study on ACEs, 47% of people experienced at least one ACE with 9% of the population having 4+ ACEs.' (Bellis et al, 2014)

Adverse events include: physical abuse, sexual abuse, emotional abuse, living with someone who abused drugs, living with someone who abused alcohol, exposure to domestic violence, living with someone who has gone to prison, living with someone with serious mental illness, losing a parent through divorce, death or abandonment.

Personality Disorder (PD)

A person with a personality disorder thinks, feels, behaves or relates to others differently from those unaffected, i.e., the average person.

The Mayo Clinic notes that those affected habitually blame others whilst finding it difficult to take responsibility. Alternatively, they find difficulty in making decisions but reject the decisions others have made.

In this concept, avoiding decisions protects identity. Criticizing the decisions that others have made, negating their behaviour, is a false reinforcement of identity.

Personality Disorder from NHS information:

> 'Borderline personality disorder (BPD) can cause a wide
> range of symptoms, which can be broadly grouped into
> four main areas (i) emotional instability – the technical
> psychological term is "affective dysregulation" (ii) disturbed
> patterns of thinking or perception – "cognitive distortions" or
> "perceptual distortions" (iii) impulsive behaviour (iv) intense
> but unstable relationships with others.'

Incidence of PD from GOV.UK:

> 'Incidence: Incidence of personality disorder and ethnicity,
> Asian 17.3%, Black 17.0, Mixed Other 16.7, White British
> 13.9, White Other 14.0.'

[In this work, the 4% difference in the incidence is an indication of the
added work for some 'ethnic' children in growing to adulthood in the
UK community.]

> 'PD following ACE: Meta-analysis of case-control studies
> showed that individuals with PD are fourteen times more
> likely to report childhood adversity than non-clinical
> control.'[26]

[As children of parents with PD have an increased susceptibility to
the disorder, there is academic debate whether it is inherited or the
result of PD parental care.]

---

[26] Porter, C., Palmier-Claus, J., Branitsky, A., Mansell, W., Warwick, H., Varese,
F., 'Childhood adversity and borderline personality disorder: a meta-analysis',
2019 DOI: 10.1111/acps.13118

CHILDREN'S VULNERABILITY TO ADVERSE EVENTS

Recapitulating the hierarchical contract and effects.

Children can become convinced that they have been responsible for untoward events in their homes and families, even events that they have not had the slightest connection with. It correlates with an unconscious rationalization that disaster has occurred because they have not fulfilled the hierarchical contract of following 'instruction'.

Sexual abuse is more disordering than less complicated adverse events. The abuser often seeks to change the hierarchical contract instructions, causes the loss of the child's benign environment, and uses the child for their own pleasure. The 'damage' is much greater if the abuser is a parent or relative or in a parental role. The only rational conclusion for the child is that they were of insufficient value to be safeguarded. The loss of self-respect often persists for life, creating susceptibility to depression and making it more difficult to establish identity.

The hierarchical contract removes both the need and the ability for children to make decisions on their own behalf. They are unable to judge the nature of an experience, so they cannot move away, cannot say 'No'.

The need to avoid responsibility for events, for deciding what happened, continues after a sexual abuse experience. They are very reluctant to recall and relate the circumstances. Sometimes, however, if a parent or apparently friendly adult suggests, 'I know it's very difficult for you to talk about this, but I think this is probably what happened', the child seizes on the narrative, as it feels like it absolves them from deciding the nature of events. Consequently, when later they are asked for details, they might happily relate the narrative supplied, often elaborating on the story, in the relief of being able to satisfy the questioner. Lawyers call it false memory syndrome.

Occasionally, in a PTSD-like response, when a child is asked to recall what happened to them, they are so inhibited that they are unable to say anything but the acute emotion the child experienced is conveyed: a synchronous feeling of terror that raises the hairs on the back of the head of an empathic therapist.

Children are disturbed and destabilized if they are coerced into making a significant decision for themselves. One boy aged eleven changed from a contented, well-adjusted boy to bad-tempered withdrawal when his parents repeatedly pressed him to decide which school he should go to. Those who have been forced into deciding which of separated parents they will live with can express bitterness about the experience for the rest of their lives.

Comment

There is what might be called a buffer zone, in that children are resilient to many mild untoward events, and they know they misbehave at times without significant or lasting effect. Negotiating the hierarchical period of mid-childhood is best managed when both child and parent fall, moderately and adaptively, into the appropriate roles.

It is a period when children should be encouraged and helped to make appropriate decisions in preparation for when they do become responsible for their own choices. Parents and carers playing board games (e.g. Monopoly) with their children can help them to understand wise and unwise choices.

Children should also be protected from events that lead to disproportionate responses. For example, in a GP's consulting room with father, mother, baby and four-year-old sibling present, a baby was given its first vaccination. This is an occasion which should be celebrated in giving the baby protection from several lethal illnesses.

Mother and father cried when their baby was being vaccinated; mother could not hold her baby or watch. Their behaviour signalled that they felt the event was one to grieve for, to separate from. As the baby 'separated' in tears, the baby would be unlikely to remember the event. Unfortunately, the four-year-old sibling would remember, and probably acquire a fear, if not a phobia, of 'the needle'.

Children need the security of knowing that the parent contains them, that any freedom they are allowed does not go as far as dangerous places. They need to know that ultimately, a parent would sooner die themselves than allow any tragedy to happen to them. Most parents understand this need and endeavour to satisfy it.

Occasionally, confidence is undermined by being used by adults in a relatively minor way. Such incidents are not uncommon, and rapidly forgotten by parents, but the parental default is an event that often remains in the child's memory. For example, many remember when they were sent to the front door to say, untruthfully, that their mother was not at home. It is a betrayal. They remember feeling that they were placed in a threatening position, made responsible for lying, when dishonesty was denigrated at other times.

In summary, the child's task is to observe and 'follow' the adult example to:
i)   discover and learn how to be socially acceptable in their family and wider tribe.
ii) gain intellectual and physical exercise, usually in school, where they also acquire the emotional intelligence to negotiate and survive in an often competitive environment.

Success in both the above can bring self-confidence, encouraged by sensibly moderate praise and respect by others that engender early self-identity.

TRANSITION AT PUBERTY, ADOLESCENCE

The radical physical changes at puberty are accompanied by an equally radical reorientation of behaviour. The hierarchical contract is lifted, adolescents become responsible for making their own decisions. It is an alternation from basic multicellular-like synchrony to unicellular-like individualism.

The most powerful sense of personal independence is found in rejection of the parents' beliefs and attitudes, in having different perceptions to what is benign or adverse and in finding new responses to events.

Many adolescents leave their families with the sense of life being a guaranteed benign environment, even one that is theirs by right. Just as the hankering to be 'master of the world' can persist from infancy, some are reluctant to be recedic, to submit to circumstances, and blame others for obstructing their progress.

The decisiveness with which some adolescents graduate from recedic mid-childhood to independence could suggest that they have no conflict about the transition. Neither would it appear that, at the other end of the spectrum, those who remain apparently contentedly at home with parents have had a conflict in making that decision.

The first group choose to define themselves through the struggle, the second group avoid the struggle, accepting clone-like roles.

A stable family with parents who have considered principles and opinions provides a workable foundation, or model, within the child, to be shaped by its own inherent personality and experiences.

In the process of differing, of distancing, from parents, it is useful if the parents have had a commitment, for example, to a sport, to religion, to university education, to increasing wealth. It provides the near adult a focus point – either to feel the parents were not as committed as they should have been and to pursue the commitment or interest more actively than the parents had done – or to have none of it, to reject it absolutely. For example, 'I hate people who play bridge' and 'I never go into a church' to 'the last thing I will ever do is to become a teacher, like Mum/Dad'. Whichever deviation is taken from that point, it is a separation from the version that the parents have handed down or it is believed that they imposed. It provides separation whilst the attributes of honesty and respect for others can be retained.

In past centuries, possibly more than the present, parents have coerced children to remain within the family, either by control or by making life excessively comfortable.

Jane Austen's 'Emma' suffered both, and repeated the behaviour in controlling others.

Children have a weak sense of identity, adolescents can have a chaotic sense of identity, of their appearance, intelligence and ability that can go from one extreme to the other in hours if not minutes. To avoid feeling worse about ourselves, our identity, we cast about for reasons and parents are easy targets.

Philip Larkin is vehement in his poem 'This Be the Verse' that parents create confusion in their children. Its creation is usually unconscious but can be deliberate for the parent's own amusement.

Parents may pass on physical, personality and behavioural attributes we would rather not have. But, without them, when consistent parenting has failed, the incipient adult is directionless, without a compass pointer. It is easily filled by the charismatic peer, the flattering adult acquaintance, the religious sect leader, political extremists and almost any other influence that floats by.

Perfect parenting is impossible. One mantra has been 'just aim to be good enough'. An alternative is 'if you are parenting a little better than you were parented, be satisfied'.

IMPOSED BEHAVIOUR

Ants, termites and honeybees 'bend' the behaviour of the whole community by confining egg, larva and pupa stages to the nest or hive. The members are diverted from any individual behaviour to a close social integration. There is an almost religious adherence to the community, they are all prepared to die in defending each other and their larvae.

We have, for centuries, used the period when species are open to becoming attached to 'break horses in', to be biddable to humans, rather than persistently independent.

With less purposeful intent, puppies are taken from their mothers when they are still immature as it encourages them to become attached to their new owners. Dogs often behave as if they are part of the family.

Two communities, African tribes and English middle/upper classes have chosen, in the past, to delegate the care of adolescent boys to mature mentors.

James George Frazer recorded in *The Golden Bough* (1890) that

African tribes sent late-adolescent boys to survive for months as a group, in the 'wild'. They were accompanied by one adult male.

In this country, boys have been sent to 'public' schools. It removes the adolescent boy striving to distance himself from the parents and lessens disaffection at home.

For both, in Africa and England, the delegated experience has been a schism, replacing the synchronous, albeit stormy, attachment to the family with a new synchrony with those with whom they survived painful challenges and deprivations, with whom they survived the 'testing period'. Consequently, like the African warriors in the film *Zulu*, like ants and bees, the junior officers in the First World War willingly allowed themselves to be sacrificed in battle.

Detachment from the family at home also removes a constructive rite of passage. For example, beating Father in a game or in other competition is a unique contribution to identity. For some fathers, this event adds to their own identity, that their son has achieved that success. For others it is an intolerable event to be avoided whenever possible – so if they formerly played chess together and it begins to look as though their child will win, there is always an excuse not to play – 'Too busy!'

* * *

Late adolescents often voice uncertainty about what they want to do or can do. There is a current preoccupation with entertainment and sports celebrities, both of which deceitfully encourage adolescents to believe any of them can achieve whatever they want to do. They ignore that random good fortune occurs, that they have been inherently physically or intellectually more able than the average. It persuades some teenagers that the only worthwhile aspiration is to achieve one form of notoriety or another. Consequently, they eschew any occupation that does not offer the possibility of stardom, the possibility of constant reinforcement of self-identity through the adulation of others.

A few, and more often their parents, are keen that they enter a profession with the potential of reinforcing self-identity and the comfort cushion of a good salary – for example, medicine.

The only certain path to identity is one we have arrived at for ourselves, but that path often begins by taking on unstimulating 'everyday' jobs, as it may be the only employment available.

When we realize we are not guaranteed a benign environment and have been able to move on from adverse circumstances in employment and in relationships, we gain confidence and resilience. Those who have never been turned down for a job or whose love has never been rejected can be less adaptable than those who have had the experiences.

A combination of circumstances can result in rebellious, socially antagonistic adolescence. Some of those who have arrived at that state find that they would like to be part of 'society' and recognize their need to change but find it impossible to impose social self-discipline. Occasionally they put themselves in a situation where the system forces hierarchical conformity, such as the Armed Services.[27]

* * *

Successful transition through mid-childhood and reconfiguration through adolescence are the foundation for a resilient identity, resilient to disaster and, less easily, to adulation.

Unfortunately, the fragilities from our behavioural evolution can, like random minefields, interrupt the process.

---

[27] One survey found that in enlisting the most undisciplined of recruits often chose to join the most disciplined Royal Marine service. Possibly an unconscious awareness that they needed others to impose a hierarchical acceptance when they could not do so themselves.

IMPERFECTIONS

There are four sources of disruption to our lives:
   The evolutionary transitions.
   The third era transformation.
   The hierarchical contract and how our society has developed.
   Anomalies categorized as psychiatric disorders.

THE EVOLUTIONARY ELEMENTS AND TRANSITIONS

Oscillation

Although oscillation is integral to and vital for cellular physiology, it carries some disadvantages. Inertia-like potential energy discourages physical exercise and seeking change, both of which contribute to our well-being.

Parallel oscillation can promote civil dysfunction in lynching and riots, personal dysfunction in 'folie a deux'.

Human growth to a stable adulthood has been founded in a childhood organized and protected by, most often, two parents in harmony. Harmony between parental couples is achieved by synchronous reciprocal (A) oscillation in sexual intercourse, initially facilitated by strong physical attraction, and second in synchronous parallel (B) rhythms in childcare and 'nest building'. An analogy could be song A and song B, both songs sung by the partners together. Unfortunately, with the passage of time, one partner wants to sing song A and the other to sing song B. Disaffection from loss of unity threatens building a life together and, more important, the harmonious parenting of children.

Potential energy prevents moving away from adverse events even after they have passed. But the most disadvantageous aspect of potential energy is that it militates against change of perceptions, of opinions. Having formed an opinion on the character of a friend, an acquaintance, media figures and organizations, including political parties, we are extremely unwilling to change our opinion and attitude. We persist with our convictions even when we are confronted with new information that would make it wiser or more rational to change.

Potential energy, change of belief, of conviction is so rare that it can, like St Paul's conversion on the road to Damascus, be called a miracle.

The rigidity is exacerbated by identity; our identity cannot help but be reduced if we are forced to acknowledge that our judgement was wrong, that we were deluded, when ability to make the 'best' decision is critical for identity. We look for reasons why we were misguided, misled, reasons to blame others for any misconceptions.

Unicellular/Multicellular Transition

Unicellular life arose 3 to 4 billion years ago, multicellular life only evolved 2 billion years later. It was possibly delayed because of the difficulty in overcoming the 'biological' need to routinely exercise separation.

Unicellular, individualistic behaviour is the default behaviour which makes social cohesion relatively fragile.

The polarized response to adverse events that arises from early organic life is to separate, move away or 'take out' the threatening intrusion, usually by ingestion. It is an elemental behaviour, and it is therefore not surprising that it surfaces in the intense competition of hominid life and even fostered cannibalism on occasions. We no longer seek to ingest those with whom we are in competition but the 'take out'/removal response is only superficially displaced by modern competitive self-identity, the acquisition of respect through achievements and occasionally destroying respect for others, a skill perfected by barristers in court.

Its sensitivity is evident when we want to protect our image of ourselves. It is very easy to interpret what is often a mild rejection as an intended insult, that it is intended to affect us, injure our identity. It causes an aggressive response; verbal aggression soon escalates into physical threat and can rapidly arouse the inherited remove or be removed attitude of our hominid ancestors.

Hierarchy

Like oscillation, hierarchy was and is necessary for physiological function. It easily gains momentum to the point that it becomes acutely addictive and in that heightened state the 'lower orders' are not experienced as a responsibility but as a nuisance or there to be used. Ultimately, both are a disadvantage to the individual 'addicted' to superiority and to those who are exploited.

Stars and famous personalities in retreat will say they were seduced by fame rather than admit they were addicted to it. It is a typical attempt to place responsibility for perceived errors elsewhere, to preserve identity.

Bias

Bias creates conflicting perceptions of events and 'best' response in the population. Those with right-wing individualistic convictions and others with left-wing 'multicellular' social convictions will always be at odds with each other.

Alternating Behaviour

The need to alternate our behaviour between recedism and apertism can provoke fluctuating erratic outbursts, impulsive actions, verbal and physical abuse of staff in airports, hospitals, etc., particularly when individuals feel they cannot move away from circumstances that are experienced (not necessarily correctly) as adverse. Although the behaviour is more common in individuals affected by personality disorder, everyone can act in that way.

THE THIRD ERA
TRANSFORMATION

INFANCY

Some infants are allowed to continue to control their lives indefinitely. One eleven-year-old's diet consisted entirely of corn flakes, large quantities of milk chocolate and several bottles of Ribena cordial in a day. In this case the control of his diet only affected his family.

In privileged circumstances, children, especially boys, have been consistently indulged throughout childhood. When that is combined with a lasting sense of entitlement to a benign environment they can destructively dominate. The children of dictators (Uday Hussein, son of Saddam Hussein) and in the past the children of princes (Henry VIII), have been 'spoilt' by having every whim satisfied. The social and material worlds are theirs to exploit, they are ruthless and intimidating to both adversaries and close friends.

GENOCIDE

Other species do not set out to obliterate adversaries. The victorious stag does not follow up his triumph by killing his defeated rival. Humans indulge in genocide without rational cause, simply 'taking out' what is experienced as just standing in the way – ultimately removing everyone else.

HUMAN INTELLIGENCE AND MEMORY

Human Intelligence and Memory have brought excessive demand upon the decision-making attribute and susceptibility to breakdown. An intelligent chimpanzee can memorize and employ a hundred symbols, the average person has a vocabulary of 25,000 to 35,000 words to interpret and decide which to use. The exceptional knowledge and intelligence brought to bear on making decisions causes susceptibility to overload and disorder.

THE WAY IN WHICH OUR SOCIETY HAS DEVELOPED

In moving away from primitive family roles, the hierarchical contract is more tenuous.

Human societies have introduced legal systems, religious beliefs and forms of monetary exchange. They have brought advantages that contribute to social cohesion and exchange between individuals but have added further demands upon our decision-making resources.

Modern Western society is hypocritical about sex. Showing a female acquaintance that she is found sexually attractive is condemned, even criminalized. At the same time fashion, cosmetics and plastic surgery heighten sexual attractiveness and behaviour. TV dramas, glamorize sexual activity. The confusing message can lead to withdrawal from society in 'incel' behaviour and, in this work, contributes to anorexia.

PSYCHIATRIC ILLNESS

Disorders categorized as psychiatric illnesses reinterpreted in the context of 'Homo imperfectus' include schizophrenia, post-traumatic stress disorder (PTSD), psychopathy, autism, attention deficit hyperactivity disorder (ADHD), anorexia, obsessive compulsive disorder (OCD), phobias, depression, mania and bipolar conditions, anxiety, personality disorder.

SCHIZOPHRENIA

The contention throughout this work has been that our acquisition of intelligence and ability to 'file' more information than other species, has resulted in susceptibility to dysfunction through overload of our decision-making facility; the dysfunction is labelled schizophrenia.

'Schizophrenia is a serious mental illness that affects how a person thinks, feels and behaves. People with schizophrenia appear to have lost touch with reality, it causes significant distress for the individual, their family members and friends. If left untreated, the symptoms of schizophrenia can be persistent and disabling.'[28]

---

[28] From National Institute of Mental Health, Mental Health Information. https://www.nimh.nih.gov/health/publications

In past decades, diagnosis and elucidation of schizophrenia has often focused on the delusions and hallucinations reported by those suffering from the condition. These unpleasant experiences can be compared to the increased physiological activity that causes a raised temperature in thyrotoxicosis and in infectious diseases: an overactivity similar to night-time dreaming in an endeavour to return the behavioural system to a balanced homeostatic state. In this work, delusions and hallucinations are largely irrelevant symptoms when compared to other features of the condition.

The following aspects of schizophrenia correlate with decision-making overload as the cause of the disorder.

Schizophrenia occurs more frequently with:

1. a) Individuals who have a high IQ. Human intelligence is founded in a shallow, low polarized, weighing of benign and adverse elements of an event that allows both to be registered simultaneously. The process can be likened to using fragile, excessively sensitive laboratory scales as opposed to more robust kitchen scales. The more sensitive a system the more susceptible to instability.

1. b) The need to resolve multiple decisions, as in divorce, in moving house, in unemployment, in moving to a foreign country or foreign culture.

2. The most significant feature of schizophrenia is that it is extremely rare, if it occurs at all, in children. Its absence in childhood correlates with children's minimal decision-making apparatus and vice versa.

3. In prolonged schizophrenia there is a burnout loss of tissue in the hind brain, the site of decision-making. It is evident in enlargement of the ventricle, an open space adjacent to the hind brain.

4. It appears to be confined to our species. We subject ourselves to many more decisions than any other mammal.

Symptoms

Sleep with dreaming reduces the emotional arousal created by events during the day; it restores the homeostatic state. The relief, the easing of emotions, by a good night's sleep is a universal experience. In the psychotic state, there is a need to recover the stability of the behavioural system. It is posited above that the need for restorative dreaming is so acute that it intrudes during waking hours in the form of hallucinations, delusions, and voices. (The possibility that the phenomena are forms of dreaming is not an original observation.) Although the hallucinations and delusions may be attempts to restore stability (like a raised temperature to restore physiological stability), it is possible that using the dreaming resource during the day disturbs the sleep rhythm at night. A disturbed sleep pattern is often an early symptom of schizophrenia.

The major symptoms of schizophrenia are separated into three formal diagnostic groups: paranoid, hebephrenic and catatonic states. They are in effect escalating forms of protection from decision-making.

Paranoid

Paranoid is commonly interpreted as 'persecution complex'. ('Paranoid' has become an abusive label, comparable to racial- or gender-demeaning epithets. Its continued use as a scientific category contributes to the stigma attached to the psychiatrically ill.)

The first elemental behaviour is defining adverse and benign environments. We all seek confidence that we have the ability to correctly define or categorize changes in the environment that could be vital to our survival. Loss of confidence in ability to make the best decision is threatening. The need to protect that confidence provokes immediate rejection of the perceptions and opinions that others introduce.

Rejecting advice, rejecting the advances of others, often aggressively expressed to emphasize the rejection, is essentially a protection of personal competence, not a persecution complex.

Hebephrenic

The hebephrenic condition is noted for its 'negative' symptom. There is little emotional expression, those who are affected by schizophrenia are withdrawn, often ceasing to wash or care for themselves. In this state, decision-making is protected by withdrawing, like a biased recedic barnacle, from exchange with others, separating from events.

Catatonia

Those with catatonic symptoms fluctuate from actively copying the words and movements of their interlocutors or others in the vicinity to virtual absence of movement. An abdication of responsibility to make any decisions.

In the severest catatonic state those affected wait for a staff member to put their arm up in a desired position, for example, for dressing, and will leave it there until it is brought down again for them.

Medication

Academically, schizophrenia and other psychiatric disorders are believed to be caused by physiological dysfunction, and anti-psychotic medication is directed to restoring cerebral biochemical processes to normality. However, the first medication that was successful in treating schizophrenia was Largactil, renowned for suppressing the rebelliousness of political prisoners. In large doses it causes a hebephrenic-like condition where the subject loses all interest in events. When there is no interest there is no stimulus to make decisions and the condition is eased. It is also relevant that many with schizophrenia are compulsive smokers; nicotine has a reputation for 'calming' the nerves, reducing any sense of urgency to make decisions.

The process of progressive deterioration in schizophrenia, in this concept, is one of:

i) overload, leading to dysfunction >

ii) leading to attempt to repair with daytime dreaming (hallucinations) >

iii) when successful returning to the same circumstances of overload >

iv) further attempt to repair >

v) repair less successful >

vi) lasting damage with loss of hind brain tissue, the ventricle or space visible on X-ray is enlarged through loss of tissue >

vii) with the damage, decision-making is weakened, less competent and therefore more susceptible to overload >

viii) system protection by avoiding every form of decision-making in a hebephrenic condition >

ix) separating from the environment, from experiencing all change, all events, catatonia.

OBSESSIVE COMPULSIVE DISORDER (OCD)

Obsessive compulsive disorder (OCD) is a common mental health condition where the individual has obsessive thoughts and compulsive behaviours.

Mid-childhood children can feel responsible for untoward events and a responsibility to prevent or correct them. That sense of responsibility for events recedes in adolescence, but like the renewal of infantile dominance in excessive hierarchy, the mid-childhood sense of responsibility can return, especially when there are factors that accentuate it: parenthood, responsibility for others' lives, and for property. An inherent predisposition also creates a susceptibility to a heightened sense of responsibility for ensuring that adverse events do not occur.

Many of us feel a need to ensure that our home is safe when we retire to sleep and satisfy that need by checking that all the doors are locked. When it is done there is a transient satisfaction and relief from responsibility. For those with either an enhanced sense of responsibility or one that has been heightened by events, the sense of responsibility persists. It can become almost impossible to satisfy, so consequently actions to avoid adverse events, to avoid loss, to avoid illness, to avoid the risk of those in our care being injured or becoming ill, are repeated compulsively again and again.

The process is reinforced when the actions are almost always successful and through the attachment of potential energy to recurrent or obsessive habits of thought and habits of action.

PHOBIAS

We are born with perception and response attributes that differ in intensity from one individual to another. There is, for example, a common aversion to the linear form of a snake and the nature of its movement. The strength of the aversion varies: it is acute for some, scarcely present in others.

The experiences that happen to us will determine whether an aversion of that nature is enhanced or diminished. The parents' attitude to snakes may be conveyed by looking at the picture of a snake with their child. 'That's a nasty animal that can kill people with a bite' will increase the child's aversion; alternatively, 'Those are interesting animals that mostly live in tropical regions, you do not find many around here' diminishes aversion.

Impressing children with the need to avoid infection and food poisoning has always run the risk of creating a phobia of possible food contamination. Urging children to avoid contact with strangers creates phobic avoidance of solitary men.

There is a current loss of a sense of protective community for children, one that is enjoyed by and an advantage for young chimpanzees. Insecurity can cause anxiety and depression amongst children; it threatened to become an epidemic through added threat from the Covid-19 pandemic. An anxious disposition can persist into adulthood.

PSYCHOPATHY

A condition defined as 'indifference to, unaware of any obligations to society, antisocial behaviour'.

In this concept, sexual reproduction or the merging of two cells could not have arisen without the ability to recognize other cells of the same species, other cells with identical oscillation. Anthropologically singing the same song.

The attribute appears to be present in the DNA of every mammalian species and like other attributes, differs in intensity between individuals. We vary between possessing a weak and a strong propensity for human synchrony. Some show a greater propensity to have synchrony with other species, for example, with dogs, cats or horses.

In our species, recognition begins soon after birth in eye-to-eye contact between mother and baby. The attribute is reinforced through infancy and into childhood by consistent physical and emotional care.

In other circumstances, when a baby is fed erratically, deprived of human contact for the first six to eight weeks of life, the vital species recognition is not animated and the ability to have empathy is lost – a psychopathic condition. When it is severe in adulthood, other humans become prey objects to be exploited, or predator objects to be neutralized.

If the baby is rescued from the damaging circumstances and given dedicated care, synchrony with others and ability to empathize may be regenerated.

AUTISM

Autism is usually diagnosed between one and three years of age. Those with autism find it more difficult to interact with other people, to understand how they think and feel. Asperger's syndrome is a mild form of the condition.

There is no certain cause, the condition is defined by its characteristics.

In this concept, those with autistic features have diminished synchronicity with others, less accord with their emotions. It can leave those affected with an increased resource in relating to other aspects of their environment, for example, to be attached to music, leading to musical ability, or having a photographic memory or mathematic skills. In effect, human emotional intelligence is partially exchanged for problem-solving IQ.

Many who research the condition are persuaded that it is genetically determined. In effect, the experiences a child has sustained or receives have no influence on the condition, it cannot be modified.

Others believe that a dramatic event, early turbulence in infancy, can initiate an autistic condition or make an inherent susceptibility to it more severe. Some children were thought to have become autistic when their fathers returned from the Second World War. In those circumstances, the mother, now expected to be a 'full-time wife', could no longer give her child the undivided interest and synchronicity that it had become used to.

Research reported in *The Times* (1 February 2022) indicates that a digital screen is not a safe substitute for interaction with mother or other carers. From the Japanese Medical Journal *Jama Pediatrics*: 'Among boys, longer screen time at one year of age was significantly associated with autism spectrum disorder at three years of age.'[29]

There is no accepted therapy that modifies the condition, but in one trial it was found that joining in synchrony, in sounds and movements, with the autistic infant led to more social engagement. It was slightly more successful when the mother allowed the child to lead the exercise.

---

[29] *JAMA Pediatr.* doi:10.1001/jamapediatrics.2021.5778 Published online 31 January 2022

ADHD

Attention deficit hyperactivity disorder is usually diagnosed at five to seven years of age and is more common in boys than girls.

In this concept ADHD is an absence of inherent hierarchy. The child is unable to accept direction, consequently unable to apply him or herself in cooperation and in learning.

Without acceptance of direction, the underlying and stronger drive is to experience change, to seek constantly renewed sensation through hyperactivity. Amphetamines and similar substances amplify sensory experiences – like satisfying hunger they reduce the need to pursue sensory stimulation. These medications are widely prescribed for ADHD and can alleviate the hyperactive element of the condition.

The emergence of autistic features at approximately three years and the later emergence of ADHD correlates with the evolutionary progression of this concept where synchrony with other cells preceded the arrival of hierarchical organization.

ANOREXIA

Anorexia is commonest in teenage girls. The condition causes particular concern in private schools. Private education arouses a belief in the pupils that their parents have chosen to pay large fees to protect them from 'danger'.

The 'danger' with the highest profile, the most grievous event, in the lives of girls and young women is that of being raped or raped and murdered.

With onset of menarche there is monthly ovulation and hormonal change. In other mammals, the hormonal arousal is often once a year or after giving birth, opening mood and physiology to coitus and conception.

It is posited that a similar hormonal effect, of greater or lesser intensity, can occur at a subconscious level in our race.

After having received expensive protection, and the reinforcement of living in a group with similar beliefs, the conflict between the greatest fear and unmanageable physiological arousal cannot be accommodated. As a male I am unable to say whether it is conscious, subconscious or both. I suspect there is slight consciousness of the conflict and a much stronger subconscious dismay. The conflict is heightened by the media and other facets of our society that can suggest the male intrusion, sex, or rape under a different name, is not only to be tolerated but welcomed.

It is difficult to live with the irreconcilable, the possibility of 'rape' cannot be removed, the hormonal cycle cannot be excised. One possible solution in the past has been to become a nun – both protected from assault and controlled. Without that religious path, the only way that some sense of management can be achieved is by controlling oneself, controlling diet.

The longer an episode of anorexia persists the more difficult it is to return to a healthy diet. In effect, the process is progressively 'engraved' until it becomes a fixed psychological and physiological existence.

The subconscious and self-controlling response of anorexia occurs in other circumstances when conflict between personal beliefs and what others want to impose, cannot be avoided. An example of this would be hunger strikes in prisons.

DEPRESSION, MANIA AND BIPOLAR CONDITIONS

It is self-evident that depression is a label for a severe persistent recedic condition; manic or restless states are labels for severe and persistent apertic modes.

There appear to be two ways in which they can become disordered.

When an overwhelming adverse event occurs, such as bereavement, it engenders a powerful recedic reaction that is not recoverable in sleep and creates a continuing, or biased, and potential-energy enhanced recedic condition.

Extremely benign events can cause a potential-energy driven apertic state. It has encouraged those who manage national lotteries to offer counselling services for those who win large sums.

Bipolar

The essential need to exercise every facility includes the rotation between recedism and apertism, a biological rhythm that is usually satisfied by our generally diurnal lives.

Since humans found how to manage and use fire, the diurnal rotation has become blurred. It was previously noted that biological rhythms can be interrupted by social and physiological events and when one rhythm is destabilized it disturbs other rhythms.

The most basic oscillatory response to change in cells is amplification of oscillation to restore stability after environmental change threatened disorder, the excessive recedic/apertic swings replicate that amplification to attempt to return the system to stability.

Bipolar disorder is considered in this work to be a biological rhythm balance disorder.

Post-Traumatic Stress Disorder

Experiences that predispose to PTSD were noted earlier in this work.

Threatening events that do not allow either recedic or apertic responses to be deployed overwhelm the decision-making facility, paralysing it.

PTSD becomes a 'marker' for the same or similar situations, a marker that is activated whenever there is any likelihood of the circumstances – the original situation – returning. The acutely uncomfortable, anxious sensations can be activated by ephemeral words, even by images that have only slight similarity to the paralysing event in a reflex-like response that shouts, 'Do not go near again.'

Anxiety

We are emotionally aroused in anticipation of significant events, of events that will be adverse or benign for us personally.

Anxiety is a mild anticipation of PTSD.

We are anxious when an approaching event requires either recedic or apertic action. If we are waiting for exam results, whether we should ready ourselves to go forward and take advantage of success or whether the result will impose recedism, a need to withdraw from the prospective event. The worst response would be paralytic failure to take either path.

In our everyday experience, an apertic mood carries with it the possibility of satisfying advantage. A recedic mood presumes loss, disadvantage. We are often anxious, whether the immediate future or the way we have behaved will make the environment benign when we can enjoy apertism or suffer the converse, adversity. A chronic anxiety state leaves those who are affected with a constant fear of the future, concern as to whether there will be adverse events, concern whether 'they have been acting wisely in preparation for tasks that arise – or not'.

The potential for feeling anxiety is accentuated in our race because failure to choose the best response is not only disadvantageous in the day-to-day management of life but also threatening to our identity.

PERSONALITY DISORDER

Personality disorder is a controversial diagnostic label, in short, whether it should be considered (i) as one or multiple diagnostic categories or (ii) as varied personality traits from the wide spectrum of human nature. It is often related to adverse events in childhood.

EPILOGUE

Neither I nor anyone else has previously followed the itinerary-like progression of evolutionary stages set out in this work. Academic colleagues will find it an amateur and naive essay.

I hoped in this work to elucidate (1) the fragile points in the system that make us susceptible to psychiatric illnesses and (2) why the characteristics of children's reaction to abuse and its unavoidable consequences are founded in childhood behavioural growth, a process that is as predetermined as physical growth to adulthood.

Both aspirations are at least partially accomplished.

In this concept I have advanced that our decision-making resource is limited and that it can be overloaded, leading to dysfunction. Many continuously add to the burden on decision-making with mobile phones. Mobile phones have created an environment where we are all continually in the same room, in 'real' time, and instant decisions can be repeatedly demanded of us. Those who are wise, filter contact.

I have also advanced in this concept that behaviour, response to change, has progressed at each stage through diminished polarization of perception and response.

In Western societies an experiment is taking place in depolarization of gender. Like other depolarizations it appears to be effected by reducing the intensity of masculinity if not of both poles, a neutering of masculine and feminine symbols.

The changing behavioural choreography makes it more difficult for adults and children to understand social behaviours and for children to begin to understand and find their way in the community, to establish a confident identity.

Depolarisation of the environment enabled intellectual growth in chimpanzees. Their increased skill reduced the challenge to survive. The loss of challenge, of change, provoked a need to find alternative stimulation and is intermittently satisfied in otherwise pointless cannibalism.

Intelligence has made humanity the dominant species on the planet but simultaneously created our susceptibility to schizophrenia.

The consequences of gender depolarisation are unforeseeable.

* * *

Finally, in returning to identity, the world is unfair, some are born with advantageous attributes. Some have better parenting. Some are given privilege.

Identity that comes from the adulation of others is longed for, is addictive, and like the air in a balloon, like alcohol, like a sugar rush, it is ephemeral.

The only identity worth having is one that we have built for ourselves.

INDEX